FIBRENETICS

Also by Gilly Smith

THE MEDITERRANEAN HEALTH DIET
(with Rowena Goldman)

Gilly Smith

FIBRENETICS

A FRESH START FOR LIFE

FOURTH ESTATE
LONDON

First published in Great Britain in 1993 by
Fourth Estate Limited
289 Westbourne Grove
London W11 2QA

A catalogue record for this book is available from the British Library.

ISBN 1–85702–158–4

Typeset by York House Typographic Ltd
Printed in Great Britain by Cox & Wyman

Illustrations by Sue Testar

CONTENTS

A Guardian Book
published as a contribution towards
the healthy eating debate

ACKNOWLEDGEMENTS

This book would never have been possible without the calming influence and encouragement of my flatmates, Wendy Lloyd and Martin Head. My editor, Jane Carr, helped me see the, wood for the trees. Kathryn Seth-Smith was the nutritionist who somehow made cellular activity and faecal mass sound interesting, and was always on the end of the phone when I needed her. Clare Davison's casual comment to me about PMS and starch prompted the delving which brought to light one of the most useful and newsworthy studies in the entire book. Nigel Barden persuaded the chefs to deliver almost on time, and their recipes prove that fibre doesn't have to be an F word, and that it's more than possible to bring together the previously estranged worlds of nutrition and cuisine.

And thanks – as always – to my agent Andrew Lownie, without whom . . .

INTRODUCTION

When the *The F-Plan Diet* came out in 1982, it became the best-selling diet in the world – probably because it encouraged us to eat as much as we wanted in the knowledge that we'd get rid of it very shortly afterwards, and more importantly because it worked. This was the first time a diet had promoted foods which helped us lose weight; in the past that had depended entirely on the calories we *didn't* eat. Deprivation seemed to be the only way to shift those extra pounds, and depression almost always came hand in hand with it. But the author of the F-Plan, Audrey Eyton, promised that we'd find slimming easier than ever before because our diet would be more satisfying and more filling than anything else we'd ever tried. We'd lose weight more quickly because a larger proportion of the calories we'd be eating would pass straight out. And what's more, we'd become really healthy and this would help keep all those life-threatening diseases like cancer and heart disease at bay. She promised that these weren't the claims of some dubious doctor but the results of a growing body of scientific evidence. She was the first person to interpret the stodgy rhetoric of the Royal College of Physicians for a lay audience. They wrote: 'It seems likely that a diet in which sugars and starches are taken in natural fibre-rich form would contribute to the control of obesity by encouraging satiety at a lower level of energy intake, and to a lesser extent by increasing the amount of potential energy lost in the faeces.' 'What that means in simple English,' wrote Eyton, 'is that if you follow a high-fibre diet, you will find that you feel more satisfied on fewer calories. And more of the calories that go into your mouth will, to put it bluntly, go straight through and down the lavatory.' Weight loss was a dead cert.

And the results were – and still are – astonishing. Sales of bran-based cereals soared by 30%, wholewheat bread by 10%, wholewheat pasta by 70% and baked beans – already very popular – by 8%; the F-Plan became the best selling non-fiction book of the year, selling millions of copies since. Up to that point, slimming books had been comparatively slow to take off, with John Yudkin's *This Slimming Business*, for example, shifting 250,000 copies over 20 years . . . By contrast, in its three weeks *The F-Plan Diet* sold 810,000 copies, matching the popularity in its day of *Lady Chatterley's Lover*.

So how is it then that ten years on we think we know all there is to know about fibre but, when push comes to shove, we're eating a third less than is recommended by experts? The answer is, amazingly, that we simply don't know what it is. Most of us still think of fibre as something to do with baked beans and unsociable dinners; bran is still something which people think they have to spoon over their food to cure a persistent bout of constipation. Ask what people think of fibre, and they'll say 'it tastes of cardboard', 'something stringy in beans' or 'sawdust stuff'. It's difficult to think of a decent recipe off the top of the head which would appeal to the foodies among us who might also want to lose weight, look and feel better and help ensure we don't end our days suffering from breast or bowel cancer. In most people's perceptions fibre is something associated with the relief of uncomfortable bouts of constipation, but not really part of our everyday lifestyle. So, where *do* you find it? How do you measure fibre intake? Is it animal, vegetable or mineral? Fibre is all a bit too confusing, difficult to find and, despite its proven health benefits, it's become a bit of an F word. *Fibrenetics* will answer all of these questions and more.

The bottom line is that we need fibre. We're suffering from an outrageous number of preventable diseases caused in part by eating too much of the wrong kinds of food. If doctors are so sure that we can cut down on heart disease and cancer, not to mention a whole host of complaints found chiefly in the West like constipation, gallstones, even piles, who are we to argue?

THE FIBRE MAN

The discovery of the relationship between fibre and diet-related diseases was largely due to the industrious examination of African stools by an English surgeon, Dr Denis Burkitt, while he was working in a teaching hospital in East Africa in the sixties and seventies.

Dr Burkitt's travels led him to some of the most remote areas of the world and slowly he began to realise that many of the diseases he'd witnessed in the West simply didn't occur there. He'd read the accounts of Dr Tom Allinson (founder of the wholemeal bread 'wi' nowt taken out') whose essays of a century ago had suggested that constipation, varicose veins and haemorrhoids could all be due to an insufficiency of fibre in the diet. Burkitt noticed that while an industry was building in Britain and America to provide laxatives to an increasingly uncomfortable public, Africans, for example, had no need for chemical assistance with their toilet activities. He made what has become a legendary comparison between the average African and Northern European stool, and concluded that our own meagre 'droppings' could be the culprit in the growing incidence of bowel cancer.

The big soft African stools which are passed in large volume became the gauge for internal health, and showed us Westerners to be the anally retentive victims of our own industrial advancement. 'The whole of the Western world is constipated,'

Burkitt told me, 20 years later, from his home in Gloucester-shire. 'There have been more changes in the way we eat in the last two hundred years than there have been in the last two thousand, and suddenly we're riddled with diseases our bodies don't know how to cope with. The Industrial Revolution was responsible for a lot of it but now that we've got so much information about where we've gone wrong, we can get back on the right track.'

Africans who lived on a rural diet of unrefined grain, fruit and vegetables, he discovered, were not suffering from the incredible rate of disease that the more affluent diet of the West seemed to be producing. Our food was becoming subjected to milling practices which positively encouraged the extraction of fibre, so little was known about its benefits. By the Second World War, vastly improved technology had heralded a new age in the availability of cheap and varied food, and nutrition-ists were more concerned that we were getting enough to eat in the wake of rationing than they were about the content of our food. White bread, refined sugar and the subsequent new industry of jams, sweets and chocolate along with hydrogen-ated fat and mass-produced meat changed the face of the British diet, and, in the process, somehow we lost sight of the whole point of eating.

AN AGE-OLD STORY

Fibre has been around since the dawn of time, and there have always been plenty of sages who propounded its health bene-fits. As early as 430BC, Hippocrates waxed lyrical about the laxative effects of wholemeal bread which he noticed was having a particularly beneficial effect on the bowels of his friends and colleagues. But it was 2,000 years before brown bread came back into favour after being dismissed as an old-

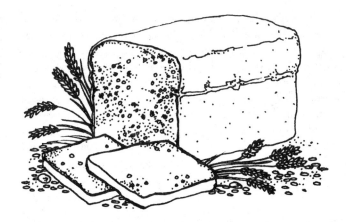

fashioned food: white bread was seen as much more sophisticated when new milling processes which refined the bran out of
bread became all the rage, despite the bubbling under of the
bran revolution at the end of the last century by the Kellogg
Brothers in the United States and Allinson in Britain.

The British diet hadn't always been so nutritionally off
course; in fact the diet of the Scots was exemplary up until
about 150 years ago. People who lived in the country areas
were stocking up on oats, barley, kale, peas, beans and lentils
and all because they were easily accessible and cheap. Living off
the land made sense, until we gave up so much of it to
industrialisation. People were much more active too. Farm-
workers in the UK 150 years ago would walk as much as 5–7
miles a day to get to work and back. The Scottish poor existed
pretty much on a staple diet of porridge and broth and while
that certainly made them regular with very low cholesterol in
the blood, it wasn't really going to inspire a generation of
aspirant youngsters to continue the diet of their forefathers.
Scotch broth with its barley, vegetables and lentils was wonderfully high in fibre but was relegated to the poorhouse as soon as

times became a little less austere. By the beginning of the new century the Western diet was taking an unprecedented turn with the dramatic change in production techniques the Industrial Revolution brought with it. There was a massive drop in the consumption of fibre from bread, cereals, oatmeal and rice, and of potatoes. Demand for luxury commodities went through the roof with chocolates, fats like butter and cream, and ice-cream among the highest climbers in the popularity charts. All of a sudden the high-fibre, low-fat diet of only a couple of decades previously had been turned upside down.

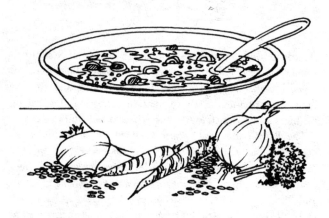

Only during the Second World War did Britons return to a more healthy diet, and this certainly wasn't through choice. Rationing of a number of foods was responsible for lower incidences of appendicitis, dental problems, obesity and diabetes. But again, with healthy food being so inextricably linked to deprivation and poverty, the nation had become conditioned to think of 'good food' as the indulgent, fatty, creamy delicacies it had spent so long going without. It was only a matter of time before we began to burst our belts and head for an epidemic of heart disease.

Of course, we shouldn't blame ourselves for our appalling inability to feed our bodies properly; our ancestors must carry the can to a certain extent. Over the last two million years, we've moved further and further away from the instinct which told us what we should and shouldn't eat. Like animals, we were once gifted with an unconscious ability to pick and choose the foods which would make our bodies more attuned to environmental pressures. Now that we don't have to rely on speed to get out of a stray mammoth's path, our bodies don't lead us directly to the source of energy. An interesting study came out of America recently in which a group of students in a controlled environment were asked to eat from a wide variety of foods. At first they went straight for meats but, over time, they gradually changed and chose more vegetables and fruits, which required less effort from the digestive system. Millions of people followed this pattern when warnings about red meat began to emerge. As we responded by cutting down on our meat intake, we began to realise how much better we felt when we ate more of a vegetarian-style diet – not to mention how much easier it was on the bank balance.

Now a new middle class has made sure that never again will they have to eat 'gruel'. Technology has told us to take it easy, to rely on gadgets to do all that heavy stuff that used to waste so much time. But most of us have been so seduced by the spoils that we didn't notice that the plug connecting mind to body got pulled somewhere along the line. We've removed ourselves so effectively from the ingredients which make up the food we eat that many of us haven't a clue how to cook even the most basic of meals. When was the last time you came in late and looked in desperation at the box of eggs, a few vegetables and cheese in the fridge and wondered what on earth to do with them? The likelihood is that you either went without or phoned for a pizza rather than whipping up a quick cheese and vegetable omelette. We're not even looking after our most basic of needs, and it's taking a visible toll on us as a nation.

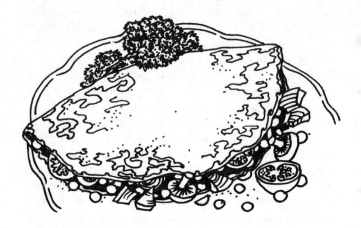

Somehow the advent of new technology didn't bother the people of Spain, Italy, Greece and the South of France whose diet is acclaimed as one of the best in the world. Not that they pay too much attention to the triumphant cries of the nutritionists who have decided that olive oil, red wine and fruit and vegetables are the key to preventing cancers and heart disease. The Mediterranean peoples have been eating the same diet for thousands of years, it's just that nobody ever bothered to ask their advice.

The plethora of goodies which grow on the fertile plains and mountains above the Mediterranean are just as rich as our own fruit and vegetables in fibre, nature's best present. Fibre doesn't conjure up quite the same exotic picture as olive oil but, in its stoic way, works just as hard to get rid of the potentially harmful substances we thoughtlessly chuck into our bodies.

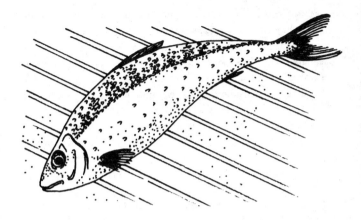

And in the same way as olive oil it encourages us to eat more interesting foods with it: so fibre opens up the larder door and lets us out of the grip of dieting.

Nutritionists have always had an uneasy relationship with people who love their food, and chefs in particular have battled with their strict guidelines on health. Nouvelle cuisine flirted with the British public in the eighties but this was no more than a passing fancy as far as the foodie who really liked to *eat* was concerned. Nutritionists claimed that moderation in all things was the best advice for the diseased and dieters alike. And as we know, moderation, in its stingy way, means having a little of what you fancy. But what if you prefer to have a large amount of what you fancy? If you're a food fan, and put eating and drinking with friends high on your list of the most pleasurable pastimes, the idea of moderation is probably anathema. This is why the Mediterranean diet with its high-fibre ingredients is so popular among foodies. The peppers they roast and marinate in garlic, herbs and olive oil, the fish steaks they grill and serve their friends on a bed of lentils, spinach, sun dried tomatoes, capers and yoghurt, and the fruits they dangle over the gaping mouths of their very best friends are not only delicious and filling but are also a great way to help prevent a variety of life-threatening diseases, not to mention an expanding waistline. Bread and pulses are widely used throughout the south of Europe, in Africa and in India where cases of heart disease and cancers are considerably lower. And these are all products which have been found on *our* home ground for centuries.

Doesn't this make you wonder why we're eating less than two-thirds of the fibre that we need? Why women are starving themselves – sometimes to death – to lose their excess weight when simply eating lots of low-fat, high-fibre foods would do it much more easily? A recent news report claimed that half the population is suffering from a condition known as TATT – Tired All The Time – yet a good breakfast can cure this instantly. Magazines are bursting at the seams with ways of patching up the effects of a bad diet using make-up and hair products. The answer has been staring us in the face all this time: a fibre-rich diet is nature's own hair care, weight loss aid and dynamiser, and packages itself better than any marketing company could ever do. Fruits, nuts, cereals and vegetables are a harvest of fibre which we've ignored for too long.

There is no more perfect machine than the human body. Imagine how magnificent it must be to be able to cope with most of the stuff we chuck into it in the course of a lifetime, and how comparatively rarely it screams for help. The liver is comparable to one of the finest laboratories money can develop; every 24 hours it filters 4,000 pints of blood, and sends out quite clear warnings when it has been over-loaded. It has an awesome ability to repair itself and, for that reason alone, it deserves some serious respect.

If we're to re-educate our eating habits and spare a thought for our insides, why not spend a bit of time reassessing our other priorities too? The Western preoccupation with squeez-

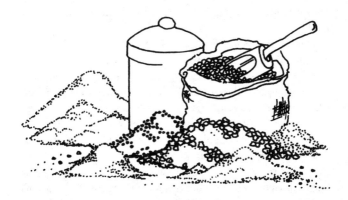

ing into unnatural shapes according to the whim of the fashion gurus has led to an obsession with eating and dieting which is becoming morally unacceptable. Not just because of the millions of war-torn, famine-ravaged people around the world who don't have that luxury but because it's a selfish pursuit which costs the National Health Service a fortune. It causes misery to millions of women who believe that they are only socially acceptable if they buy a size 10, and it nurtures a society hellbent on making any well-adjusted individual feel guilty about their love handles.

One of the most important issues – particularly for women – to emerge from this book is that eating badly seems to come down to low self-esteem. Women are often very good at giving themselves a hard time and food, along with its essential minerals and vitamins, is often one of the first casualties. Slimming is in many cases about much more than just wanting to be thinner, but the turning point can come from the understanding that eating properly *does* help you lose weight. The recipes at the back of the book are low in fat and high in fibre, and should do more to convince slimmers to welcome food back into their world than all the diet books on the market ever could.

The adage 'a healthy mind is a healthy body' may be hackneyed, but the wide variety of studies mentioned in this book which cover everything from skipping breakfast to abnormal toilet habits all send out the same message – eat and the world smiles with you, diet and you're on your own. Experts have spent a fortune researching these studies, and seem to be crystal clear about the main role of fibre in the diet: eating low-fat, high-fibre foods *does* reduce the risk of many of the most common diseases in the Western world; it *does* help us reach the right weight for our height, and it really *does* make us feel better about ourselves. So if you've been starting your day with a cigarette and a cup of black coffee, and going to work on an empty stomach, spare a thought for your colon where many of the nastiest diseases breed. You wouldn't go to work without cleaning your teeth, would you? So give your insides a sweep out, too, with a high-fibre breakfast. One in three people in Britain will suffer from cancer at some time in their lives, and changing your eating habits to a low-fat, high-fibre diet could help protect *you* from the disease.

Think how much time we'd have to concentrate on more interesting things if we weren't worrying about our figures. Ask your friends and partners how interesting it is to hear you harping on about your diet all the time, how much fun it is to go out to eat with someone who's counting calories. Chapter by chapter, *Fibrenetics* will tell you just how easy it is to eat enough fibre to look and feel better, and to finally kick the whole concept of dieting out the window. It will show you around the diet-related Western diseases and the most challenging of the holistic health treatments. Finally, the recipes in The Beanfeast (p. 147) from some great chefs will close the last chapter of your old eating regime and open the first of your fresh start for life.

ONE

FIBRE FACTS

Picture the harvest festivals of your childhood. Plaited breads, corn dollies and sacks of oats and barley in the church hall, surrounded by sheaves of wheat, apples, pears, cauliflowers, cabbages and other food from the land. This is where you'll find your fibre: in the nuts, grains, fruits and vegetables which are the key to better health, greater vitality and looking as good as you can. Apart from the church communities in this country, we've more or less given up giving thanks for our harvest, but the Americans still grandly reckon that a pumpkin represents the kind of natural goodness their nation was built upon, and feast on some of the best of it on their Thanksgiving Day.

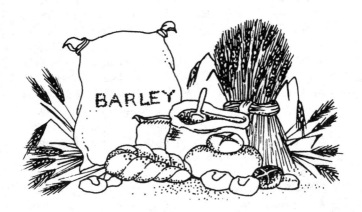

FIBRENETICS

Fibre has always been seen as a straightforward kind of food. Its image hasn't exactly been sexy; ask most people what they think of fibre, and they'll tell you that it's something to do with going to the toilet a lot. But a wealth of fascinating new evidence has confirmed that it is no less than a warrior against an endless list of life-threatening diseases: possibly more than any other food group, fibre is the most important in maintaining the body's natural defence system. With its help, our bodies can stand guard against the toxins or poisons frolicking in some of the foods we eat, simply and effectively pushing them out of our systems as waste.

Fibre is the key to liberating us from our obsession with food. At the moment many of us are dictated to by hunger pangs – the result of low levels of sugar in the blood. Eating enough fibre regulates these levels and ensures that we don't go through the constant cycle of craving followed by guilt that haunts millions of us throughout the day. Mid-morning chocolate and a desperate need for an afternoon kip will become things of the past. Imagine how much more energy you'll have at work and at play. The weight you've been trying to get rid of for years will steadily fall off and your body will gradually find the level it's happy with. Constipation won't be an occasional hassle or a never-ending nightmare any more, and foreign business trips which have always been a bit of a bummer as far as keeping regular is concerned will become something to look forward to. Diverticular disease, irritable bowel syndrome and even bowel cancer will cease to trouble so many of us, and the threat of heart disease as we reach our forties will no longer hang over us so menacingly.

Too good to be true? This chapter sets out to tell you exactly what this much maligned cure for everything from dull hair to a dodgy metabolism is all about. If it really is the key to an easy, healthy new start then we need to know how to find it, and how much of it to eat.

WHAT IS FIBRE?

Fibre is a type of carbohydrate which remains intact in the intestine. It comes from the indigestible part of plants which forms their backbone – the skins of sweetcorn and beans, the cellulose fibres which you can see forming the web in the leaves of your greens. It comes in two types, soluble and insoluble – the first is soft and mushy, the second coarse and hard. Kidney beans, for example, are rich in soluble fibre while wheat-bran is rich in insoluble fibre. Soluble fibre is also found in other pulses as well as fruit and vegetables, oatbran and barley. It dissolves in water and becomes a gummy substance in the stomach which gives a feeling of being full while delaying the absorption of sugar and other nutrients.

Soluble fibre is more important in the upper gut where it can slow the digestive and absorption processes. That means that time can be given for all the nutrients of a good meal to get into the bloodstream. If we don't eat enough fibre, our blood glucose levels, which keep the body ticking over, may fluctuate drastically. One minute we'll have no appetite at all, the next we'll crave some sweets so intensely that we can't concentrate properly. As what goes up must come down, we soon find our blood sugar plummeting well below the levels the body needs in order to function properly. These peaks and troughs are to be avoided. We always come down after the high, feeling irrational and tired.

These are clear messages from your body to your brain to get its act together. The slower and more regulated absorption of glucose into the bloodstream, which a regular fibre intake ensures, means an end to those cravings which send us running to the sweet shop for a chocolate fix. A steadier stream of glucose also means more constant energy levels and fewer hunger pangs throughout the day, which is a godsend for people who want to lose weight and for those who want to stay awake and alert for important meetings.

The other type of fibre, which provides the central theme of *Fibrenetics*, is insoluble fibre, mainly found in wholegrain cereal, and its job is to add bulk to the faeces by absorbing water and then propelling them out of the body. Nutritionists have called it nature's broom because of its ability to sweep the system clean of any unhealthy elements which would otherwise lurk in the intestine, causing a wide variety of problems from constipation to cancer. The ability of insoluble fibre to remain undigested once it has been eaten was what alerted Audrey Eyton to the concept of the F-Plan diet. 'If you're indelicate like I am, and peer down the loo,' she explained, 'you'll see that there's a lot of sweetcorn in your stools – if you eat sweetcorn that is – along with other foods high in fibre like peas and beans.' If it was passing straight out in its original form, it couldn't be taking with it anything the body needed, she suspected. And if there was a food which was so super-efficient, she wanted to know about it.

You might think that if fibre is playing the role of a vacuum cleaner, and emptying its bag out into your loo, it won't be leaving much in the way of nutrients for the body to feed off. But the nutrients of a fibre-packed food like wholemeal grainy bread for example are in the bread rather than the fibre. Bread and cereals will give you a heady cocktail of vitamins B1 and B3, and minerals like calcium, magnesium, sodium, iron, selenium and zinc. While the body hives these away into the bloodstream, the fibre heads straight down to the colon to absorb all the waste that the body doesn't need. When it's done its job, it will stay in the faecal mass which is heading towards your lavatory pan, and should you choose to have a look, you'll see that this turbo-charged vacuum cleaner is in fact nothing more than a few husks of wheat.

Unlike the other carbohydrates that it comes wrapped in, fibre provides virtually no actual energy for the body to burn up. Potatoes, pasta and rice do contain calories, but carbohydrates are easier to burn off than fats. The Department of Health recommends that we eat about 18g of fibre per day; that's a bowl of All-Bran for breakfast with some wholemeal toast, a jacket potato with broccoli, spinach or any leafy greens for lunch and an orange, apple or pear – or all three – at some point in the day. Not exactly difficult to achieve, but our fibre intake is still too low; on average we eat a third less than we should with 75% of men and 94% of women consuming less than the targets set by the Department of Health, even though a bowl of All-Bran can give us half our daily requirement. The reason men tend to eat more fibre is probably to do with the terror that many women still have of the humble potato and its starchy fellow food-group members. In the pursuit of the perfect body, women tend to miss breakfast and hold up the sign of the Cross at any carbohydrate, but evidence overwhelmingly shows that depriving yourself of these essential foods just does not work in the weight war. A diet packed with carbohydrates will burn off any excess you've been carrying around on your hips, while at the same time arming your body's defence system for its attack on disease.

But how much do we know about where to find fibre? Which of the following types of bread for example – wholemeal, brown, Hovis or white – has the most fibre? The answer is wholemeal, with white coming in last. If that seems too obvious, try this little test to see how much you really know about fibre. We all know that All-Bran is high in fibre – at 9.6g per serving it makes up more than half the recommended fibre

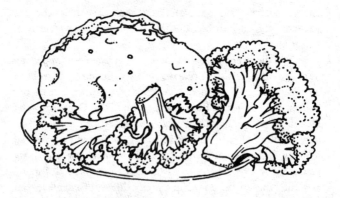

quota for the day. But what about other foods such as biscuits, fruit and vegetables? The Department of Health tell us we need 18g of fibre a day, but in this country we lag badly behind, getting around 12g in our daily food intake.

WHERE DO YOU FIND YOUR FIBRE?

PULSES AND BEANS

These are the seeds of the legume family and are of the water-soluble fibre type. They contain enormous quantities of protein and are an essential part of a vegetarian's diet. But the poor old bean has had a hard time fighting its image as flatulence food which takes forever to soak in advance, and could kill you if you don't boil it for long enough. The truth is that while you should soak some pulses overnight before cooking, there are plenty of beans – kidney, baked and haricot, for example – which come ready soaked, cooked and drained in cans. The dried versions, if cooked properly – simmered for 20–30 minutes until soft – won't cause flatulence unless you eat too much of them and too often. Take a tip from master chef

---

FIBRE FINDER

1. How do you think the fibre content of peanuts compares with that of walnuts?
2. If carrots come in at 1.5g per 60g serving how does a plate of baked beans fare?
3. Which has the higher fibre content – dried figs or dried dates?
4. If frozen peas have 3.3g of fibre, how much do canned peas have?
5. Will you get more fibre from an oatcake or a portion of Brussels sprouts?

Answers
1. peanuts 1.6g; walnuts 0.9g
2. 5g
3. figs 1.5g; dates 0.5g
4. 4.1g
5. oatcake 0.8g; Brussels sprouts 2.8g

Raymond Blanc's cookbook and add a smattering of fresh grated ginger to lentils and pulses to reduce any gases; they'll taste wonderful too. Theories abound as to how spices work, and while scientists concentrate on the more obvious food groups in their fight against cancer most of the legendary power of spices remains relegated to folklore. Ginger has, however, been shown to help relieve seasickness, ulcers and rheumatoid arthritis as well as flatulence. We know that it is a powerful anti-oxidant, helping our body's natural defence system to fight off carcinogens (cancer-causing substances). It is a powerful blood thinner, and is even thought to work as an antibiotic, especially effective against the salmonella bacteria which can be present in eggs and chicken.

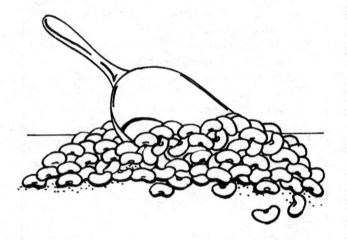

FRUIT AND VEGETABLES

The skins of fruit and vegetables are particularly rich in fibre. Obviously that doesn't mean eating banana and melon skins, but don't peel apples and pears and deny yourself all that goodness. Evidence is piling up to show that a vegetarian diet is much better for us; experts believe that the risk of cancers of the breast, bowel or colorectum, pancreas, larynx, lung and stomach can all be reduced by a much higher intake of just about every fruit and vegetable nature provides.

One of the very first studies into the benefits of vegetarianism was carried out in the fifth century when Daniel asked King Nebuchadnezzar, the ruler of ancient Babylon, to perform an experiment to see how much influence diet had on looks. 'Submit us to this test for ten days,' Daniel said. 'Give us only vegetables to eat and water to drink; then compare our looks with those of the young men who have lived on the food assigned by the king.' According to the Bible's book of Daniel (1: 11–16) this duly happened, and at the end of the ten days, the veg-eaters looked healthier and better nourished than their younger colleagues. Not exactly scientific evidence perhaps, but vegetarians will swear that they were definitely on the right track.

BRAN

Bran is one of the richest sources of fibre, and also provides many nutrients. It is the outer coating on cereals, for example the husk of wheatgrain, and is only really found in extracted form. White flour has been so refined that all the bran will have disappeared, so try to buy the wholemeal version. Bran is readily available as an ingredient in breakfast cereals – there are plenty of varieties on the market, and if you avoid those high in fat, you'll be giving your body a huge boost.

BROWN RICE AND WHOLEWHEAT PASTA

The fibre-packed husks of rice can either be thrown away in the processing of white rice or kept intact as brown rice and sold in health shops and on the top shelves of supermarkets. Brown rice has always had a bad image, and the reason is that enemy of the twentieth century – time. White rice, with husks removed, takes less than 11 minutes to cook, while brown – husks and all – rice can take more than 30 minutes. The same applies to wholewheat pasta, although it doesn't take quite so long. Try varying your pasta and rice so that now and again,

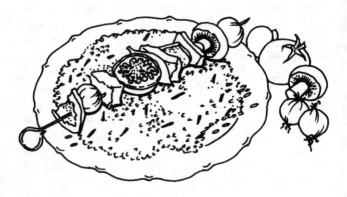

when you *can* find the time, you treat yourself to the stuff that nature intended us to enjoy.

WHOLEMEAL BREAD

Denis Burkitt, the man who made fibre a household name, suggests that we eat five pieces of wholemeal bread a day to boost our levels of fibre. The nutty, grainy brands can make every difference to an otherwise dull sandwich, and are easily obtainable these days.

A NOTE ON WHEAT INTOLERANCE

Many people are finding that they have an intolerance for wheat, and are confused as to how something which is supposed to be so beneficial should be so harmful to them. If you suspect you might have an intolerance to wheat, you'd be wise to consult your doctor for advice.

Because fibre is found in the cell walls of plants it has a very rigid architecture and takes a bit more chewing than other foods, all of which is good news for people who are overweight and don't want to be. As well as releasing the enzymes which we need for digestion, the longer we chew, the more full up we feel, and the less likely we are to snack through the day. 'Grazing' on lots of fruit and vegetables throughout the day is supposed to be the best way of keeping energy levels consistent and boosting fibre intake. But British and Americans are notoriously bad grazers, preferring instead to eat large meals three times a day. By overloading the system like this, we tend to feel like a lie down after eating, rather than feeling refuelled and ready for action. But the idea of eating smaller meals more often could be one of the most important issues to emerge in the understanding of obesity, cancer and even premenstrual syndrome.

NIBBLERS V. GORGERS

A Canadian study recently looked into the benefits of grazing and found that the test group of men who ate 17 snacks per day were in better shape than those who ate three full meals a day instead. The Nibbling versus Gorging study at the University of Toronto discovered that nibbling reduced cholesterol in their all-male subjects, and released a more constant stream of glucose into the bloodstream. The nibblers urinated more, and reduced their insulin levels; they were never hungry while the gorgers found their blood-sugar levels dropping between meals and needed to be boosted by snacks.

The study was designed to look at the benefits of grazing on diabetics and obese patients, and aimed to find out if different eating regimes could influence a change in metabolism. There was reason to believe that eating meals less frequently – one or

FIBRE CONTENT OF EVERYDAY FOODS

Serving size (grams)	Fibre content (grams)	BREAD
25	1.5	Wholemeal
25	0.9	Brown
25	0.8	Hovis
25	0.4	White

FLOUR

Serving size (grams)	Fibre content (grams)	
25	2.3	Wholemeal
25	1.6	Brown flour
25	0.8	White flour
25	1.7	Oatmeal – raw
25	0.5	Rice – brown

NUTS

Serving size (grams)	Fibre content (grams)	
25	1.9	Almonds
25	1.1	Brazils
25	1.1	Chestnuts
25	1.6	Hazelnuts
25	1.8	Coconut
25	1.6	Peanuts
25	1.4	Peanut-butter
25	0.9	Walnuts

BRAKFAST CEREALS

Serving size (grams)	Fibre content (grams)	
40	9.6	All-Bran
40	8.8	Bran Buds
30	3.9	Bran Flakes
30	3.0	Sultana Bran
30	2.1	Fruit 'n Fibre
30	1.8	Country Store
30	2.7	Raisin Splitz
30	2.7	Summer Orchard
30	0.3	Corn Flakes
40	2.6	Muesli

BISCUITS & PASTRY

Serving size (grams)	Fibre content (grams)	
25	2.9	Crispbread - rye
12	0.3	Digestive
12	0.2	Gingernuts
25	1.5	Oatcakes
25	0.5	Shortbread
50	1.1	Short pastry

RICE

Serving size (grams)	Fibre content (grams)	
150	1.2	Brown

Serving size	Fibre content		Serving size	Fibre content	
		VEGETABLES			**FRUIT** (raw)
75	1.9	Carrots	100	1.8	Eating apples
75	1.9	Beetroot	75	2.6	Avocado Pear
75	2.6	Swedes	100	1.1	Banana
100	1.4	Potatoes – jacket	100	3.1	Blackberries
100	1.1	Potatoes – new	100	0.9	Cherries
100	1.2	Potatoes – peeled & boiled	15	0.5	Dates – dried
100	1.6	Spinach	20	1.5	Figs – dried
100	3.0	Broccoli Tops	100	0.7	Black Grapes
100	3.6	Spring Greens	80	1.0	Grapefruit
100	4.8	Sprouts	150	1.5	Melon
90	1.6	Cabbage	160	2.7	Orange
90	2.2	Cabbage – raw	110	1.7	Peach
90	1.4	Cauliflour	170	3.7	Pear
30	0.3	Celery – raw	24	0.5	Raisins
80	1.4	Leeks	60	1.5	Raspberries
30	0.3	Lettuce	100	1.1	Strawnberries
65	3.3	Peas – frozen	24	0.5	Sultanas
85	4.1	Peas – canned	80	1.0	Pineapple
65	2.9	Peas – fresh			
120	7.8	Broad beans			**FRUIT**
60	2.8	Butter beans			(cooked with sugar)
135	5.0	Baked beans			
90	1.7	Runner beans	140	3.9	Blackcurrants
90	3.7	French beans	140	2.7	Gooseberries
120	2.3	Lentils – split	140	1.7	Plums
125	1.6	Corn-on-the-cob	24	0.6	Prunes
60	0.8	Sweetcorn – can	140	1.7	Rhubarb
85	0.9	Tomatoes – raw			
60	1.0	Onions			

two a day rather than lots of snacks throughout the day – was responsible for a higher risk of cardiovascular disease. This theory was only recently confirmed because earlier studies were thwarted by the inability of the very overweight subjects to cut down on their portion sizes. As a result of being encouraged to eat more often, they put on even more weight because their total calorie count was suddenly so high. In the Toronto study, scientists were able to control the subjects' nibbling and found that eating three main meals rather than snacking *could* contribute to obesity.

The mind-over-matter camp of hypnotherapists who work with slimmers agree that nibbling works better on the subconscious level. The Farago Clinic in North London equips its patients with a few weight-loss techniques including self-hypnosis coupled with the golden diet rule of nibbling. Robert Farago agrees that eating small but regular amounts through the day will keep your glucose levels stable and stop you feeling ravenous at the end of the day. 'Hunger is one of our deepest subconscious urges,' he explains. 'When your blood-sugar levels fall too low, the subconscious message to eat gets magnified – and you end up overeating.'

Nibbling is an art which, if you can keep your portions to a reasonable size, has been proved to help prevent heart disease, weight gain and to keep energy levels consistent. But beware of the hundreds of psychological motivations for eating disorders, and put the studies into your own personal context. If you think you have an eating problem look into your head first and your larder second . . .

FIBRE AND PREMENSTRUAL SYNDROME (PMS)

'Nibbling' can also help to relieve PMS, the nightmare of irrational behaviour, tearfulness and bloating that precedes

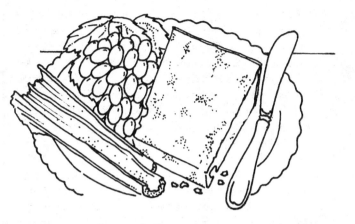

millions of women's periods. Evidence for this has emerged recently despite the extraordinary claims made by a group of psychologists at the British Psychological Society conference in 1993: Dr Priscilla Choy, a lecturer in health and psychology at Nottingham University, said PMS is *all in the mind*. Dr John Richardson of Brunel University agreed with her assertion that it is all a myth, adding that depression is unconnected to the menstrual cycle. 'I don't believe it exists as a clinical entity,' he said. Dr John Bancroft, head of the medical research council at Edinburgh, said premenstrual tension had more to do with being neurotic or depressed and that it is more often connected with personality, emotional difficulties and depressive illness.

Even some female newspaper columnists stood by them; Linda Lee Potter of the *Daily Mail* said on Radio 4's Midweek that PMS was in the mind and that if women felt a bit weepy before their period, they should just stay out of people's way and get on with their work. This stiff-upper-lipped message was received with a snarl of outrage and disbelief by most women. It doesn't help when very real problems are dismissed and, seeming to contradict these unsympathetic claims, a recent

Woman's Own survey reported that nine out of ten women suffer from PMS and one in three take time off work because of it; 85% complained of irritability, 72% of tearfulness, 61% of tiredness and 68% crave chocolate; 28% go off sex, 26% get no sympathy from their partners and worryingly 76% reported that it gets worse as we get older.

Luckily, scientists have responded too and have given clear, easy ways to deal with what does continue to seem like a very real complaint; once again, food seems to be the answer. Recent research shows that PMS can be a thing of the past if we eat enough starch at regular intervals. Fibre is found in the same foods as starch (which is another form of carbohydrate), giving your PMS a double whammy as they both regulate the level of glucose in the blood, limiting the peaks and troughs which cause the cravings, irritability and anxiety. But more importantly, perhaps, fibre also expels the extra oestrogen which can be produced in sufferers, through the faeces.

A WOMAN'S GUIDE TO HER OWN BODY

In order to understand how it all works, we have to get to grips with what happens inside our bodies every month. The fact that most of us haven't a clue reflects how little attention we pay to the frantic messages our bodies are sending us. If a pre-menstrual women is suffering from swollen breasts, a chocolate fixation and is on the verge of stabbing her perfectly genial partner, you'd think she'd realise that her body was trying to tell her something. So here's the laywoman's guide to hormones, periods and monthly hell.

Ordinarily, oestrogen is produced by the ovaries to make sure that the lining of the womb is kept healthy and to thicken it during the premenstrual period. After 8–10 days, the ovary releases an egg and secretes another hormone called progesterone. If the egg isn't fertilised progesterone levels normally then decline. Their reduction causes the lining of the uterus to be shed and we get a period.

Meanwhile the blood is pumping the oestrogen around the body, down to the colon and reabsorbing it back into the blood. All fine and dandy if we're producing the right levels of oestrogen. If we're not, levels can be wildly off balance when they go back into the bloodstream. By eating a good amount of fibre in our diet, these extra levels can be prevented from being reabsorbed into the blood by the mass of waste collecting in the colon. Fibre sweeps the whole lot up into a big bundle, and that extra oestrogen is then simply expelled in the faeces with all the other waste.

Progesterone depends entirely on the normal action of oestrogen; if oestrogen is out of control, the body will underproduce the progesterone hormone – the cause of a lot of PMS symptoms. Dr Katherina Dalton from the Premenstrual Syndrome clinic at University College Hospital in London and Wendy Holton of PMS Help recently found that women who were asking for help for PMS were leaving very long gaps between meals. They concluded that this had a great deal to do with the erratic behaviour that characterises PMS. They explained in their report that, following a *large* meal, there's a significant increase in metabolic activity in order to send all the different nutrients on their way to do their various jobs. Dalton and Holton therefore recommend eating lighter meals at three-hourly intervals to keep the blood glucose steady.

Some experts think that women who suffer particularly badly from PMS tend not to eat enough fibre and B vitamins, found in foods such as spinach, green beans, cereals and bananas.

But premenstrual tension cannot simply be dismissed by telling women to eat their greens; scientists have found that they can divide sufferers into sub-groups.

THE PRE-MENSTRUAL TENSION BREAKDOWN

PMT-A is the premenstrual anxiety, irritability and nervous tension which most women experience; if you find yourself storming through the supermarket just before your period and verbally attacking an assistant for hiding the tampons, you probably fall into this category. Elevated blood oestrogen and low progesterone have been observed in PMT-A women. Eating more of vitamin B6, found in fibre-filled foods like wholegrains, cereals, potatoes, nuts, and greens, as well as fatty fish, egg yolk, and bananas, seems to reduce these symptoms.

PMT-B is associated with water retention, bloating and weight gain. Again, vitamin B6 will bring down levels of the hormone aldosterone which is causing the problem. This is the second most common sub-group of premenstrual sufferers. Women who have particularly sore and swollen breasts before their period will also benefit from the extra vitamin E found in seeds, wholegrains, greens, egg yolk and vegetable oil. Salt should be cut right down to discourage the water retention that salt causes with or without PMT. Just to make matters worse, even though you're not urinating effectively, on the very few occasions that you do manage to pass water, you're also passing essential magnesium thanks to the action of the wild aldosterone hormone. Increasing your intake of leafy greens, pulses, nuts and shellfish is the best to beat this. And a word of warning: *don't* take diuretics. They'll deplete your magnesium and then your body will really start to take it out on you.

PMT-C is characterised by a craving for sweets, increased appetite and indulgence in refined sugars. This can be followed by palpitations, fatigue, fainting spells, headaches and the shakes. Magnesium helps here too, and you'll find this in bread, pulses, nuts, shellfish and milk. These sub-groups may help scientists to categorise their female subjects but if you suffer from all three, *boy* do you need some fibre.

Finally, PMT-D is the least common but most dangerous and is characterised by deep depression, withdrawal, insomnia, forgetfulness and confusion that leads to real misery for thousands of women. Sufferers complain of being lethargic, incoherent and having trouble verbalising. They don't normally complain or seek medical advice on their own but are brought to a psychiatrist by a friend or a relative. Suicide, murder and arson can be the extreme results of PMT-D. Scientists found that oestrogen and progesterone in a group of PMT-D women's blood were at abnormal levels during the premenstrual week. The former was lower than normal, and the latter higher. The scientists, worried that changes in diet weren't going to be enough to help these women, recommended therapy.

This was the advice 46-year-old Barbara Moss received when she tried to get help for her appalling premenstrual tension before she discovered a way of curing herself. She found that by eating any starchy food every couple of hours, she managed to stop the endless cycle of rage and tantrums followed by guilt and despair, not to mention the bloating which left her with incredibly painful breasts. She had been eating three meals a day, and hadn't really bothered with carbohydrates. Now she makes sure that she has cereal and toast for breakfast and crisps, Ryvitas or digestive biscuits for a mid-morning snack followed by a sandwich for lunch. In the afternoon, she'll snack again on biscuits or crisps and in the evening eat a jacket potato, pasta or rice with her meal. She can have anything she likes with them, but she must have the carbohydrates if she's to avoid PMS.

This starch diet has been endorsed by Dr Dalton and Wendy Holton whose PMS clinics and support group take them to the frontline of this monthly battle for millions of women. Grazing throughout the day, they agree, will regulate the all-important blood-glucose levels. Extra oestrogen will also then be able to pass out of the body in the faecal mass which fibre helps to build up.

THE STARCH DIET

Holton and Dalton recommend eating a high-fibre breakfast within 30 minutes of getting up, a baked potato or sandwich with a low-fat filling at around 1 p.m., a banana or a couple of digestive or rich tea biscuits mid-afternoon, and a sandwich before dinner. Pasta with meat or fish and plenty of vegetables should be eaten early enough for you to digest it fully before going to bed, and they even recommend more starch such as crispbreads or crisps as a late supper.

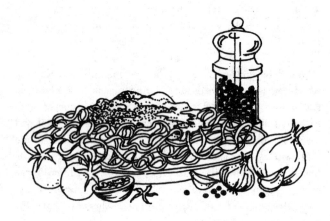

For Barbara Moss, the diet has been a life-saver. Before she chanced upon it her glucose levels were plummeting as she reached for another chocolate bar, and rocketing sky high as she devoured it. She told me that she had lost weight on her

starch diet so far, but she'll need to replace some of those crisps
and biscuits with bread, pasta or potatoes if she wants to look
after her long-term health. The fats in the foods we eat are
major contributors to heart disease in biscuit-bingeing Britain.
She says that she has learnt to listen to her body's cravings more
carefully, and realises, for example, that it's not that she has a
particular soft spot for bananas, but that her body *needs* the
vitamin B6 they give her.

Barbara's story is common to millions of women; she can't
believe how her husband managed to stick with her as, month
after month, she flew into violent and totally irrational rages. In
the search for a cure she had been referred to a clinical
psychologist, prescribed Valium and dismissed as a hysterical
woman before she realised that her body was screaming at her
to feed it properly. 'The first time that I didn't start flaring up
for no apparent reason just before my period,' she told me, 'I
burst into tears anyway – out of relief.'

The higher level of oestrogen in the blood is also one of the
contributory factors in the development of breast cancer, so by
including more fibre in your diet to alleviate your PMS you
could also be helping to insure yourself against one of the
biggest killers in Britain. Again, allowing fibre to prevent the
reabsorption of the extra oestrogen when it gets to the colon
means that it can't do any damage.

Breast cancer affects one in 12 women in Britain, and causes
14,000 deaths per year. And, worryingly, experts predict that it
will increase across Southern and Eastern Europe as trends in
their eating and working habits become more like our own.
High-fat products in particular are the kind of foods which are
associated with affluence, so as more populations become
exposed to our eating patterns in the richer West and copy

them they could start to suffer from the same kind of diseases which are currently in the minority in their own countries but are killing us in the West.

If only they would realise that they're on to a good thing. Already the younger Italians, Spaniards and Greeks, more susceptible to advertising than their grandparents, think it's trendy to dismiss olive oil as granny food. Yet the traditional natural foods of the Mediterranean countries make up what experts have agreed is one of the best diets in the world.

AN ILL WIND

For many people, the burning issue about fibre is flatulence. Tell friends your discovery about fibre and weight loss, not to mention how you've found a way of keeping your energy levels regular, and cancer and heart disease at bay by eating fibre, and they will probably keep out of your way for a couple of weeks. Increasing your fibre intake suddenly *can* give you wind, but your body will adapt in no time at all – within two or three days, the problem will have disappeared completely. Ask any vegetarian who relies on pulses for proteins about the problem and you'll find that the flatulence fallacy is no more than a lot of hot air.

After those two or three days of stomach rumbles, constipation will become a thing of the past, especially if you're drinking a lot of water. Fibre works by absorbing water which then pushes the body's waste out quickly and effectively. We should be drinking at least eight glasses per day; keep a bottle of water in the fridge or on your desk and sip from it throughout the day. It's cheaper and better for you than an endless supply of canned drinks, less of a fix than tea or coffee, and you'll be more aware of how much you're drinking. You should be getting through a 1.5 litre bottle every day.

FAT FIGURES

The Department of Health is probably more vociferous about the need to cut down on fat than it is about upping our fibre intake. Eight out of ten of us are still eating too much fat but cutting down, changing to a more Mediterranean style of diet and eating real food rather than convenience shrink-wrapped TV dinners will may include a much higher intake of fibre.

In a recent survey 58% of people didn't realise that pasta is low in fat, 45% didn't know that breakfast cereals are low in fat, and 68% of people were under the mistaken impression that avocado pears are low in fat. The truth is simple – fat is fattening if you eat too much of it, but learn to use it wisely and you could find yourself forgetting about calorie counting for ever. Choosing a fat that's low in saturates and high in poly-unsaturates or monounsaturates such as olive oil or vegetable oil for cooking, and also grilling, baking or boiling, will open up new avenues in eating. That 115g rump steak you used to fry gives about 15g of fat but when grilled comes down to only 7g if all the visible fat has been cut off.

Starchy carbohydrates like rice, potatoes and cereals are easily burnt off, and we can eat twice as much of them as foods that are high in fat and still get the same calories. It's a happy medical fact that we can lose weight by eating more of the filling carbohydrates. The potato and the pasta twirl have been wrongly accused for too long of being major enemies in the weight war but, with expert reports pouring out of the wood-work, they're finally taking their rightful position again at the top of the nutritionist's list of goodies.

THE VIEW FROM INSIDE

It's hardly surprising that we abuse our bodies so much considering how little we actually know about the digestive process.
You might remember fragments of your biology lessons but,
like the majority of us, you'll find it hard to apply them to your
own eating patterns. All good diets are based on knowing how
the body works.

Today's nutritionists might question the Hay diet which has
been around for nearly a century. Its creator, Dr William
Howard Hay, believed that his overweight body and diseased
heart functioned better if they weren't fed starches and proteins
at the same time. That's not to say he thought that we should
exclude either from our diet, but because the body metabolises
different food groups at varying speeds, he believed it was too
much to ask the body to deal with them all at once. In short, not
all the goodness that food provides is being extracted before it
is being passed on its way if you eat it all together. He reckoned
that you shouldn't even have fruit as a dessert after a meal of
carbohydrates or proteins. While this may be true, people who
stick to the Hay diet tend to be those who have severe illnesses
or disabilities, and have little option other than to make such a
radical change to their eating habits.

Philip Owens, the 32-year-old chef at Leicester Square's Arts
Theatre Café in London, is one such person. At 30, he was two
stone heavier than he is now and virtually crippled with
arthritis. His blood supply was not reaching his legs due to a
condition called avascular necrosis and this was causing his
bone to die off. He felt he had no choice other than to look at
his diet. His cooking is based on rustic Sicilian cuisine which
contains olive oil rather than butter, so cutting out dairy
products was easy enough. Relying on vegetables and pasta or

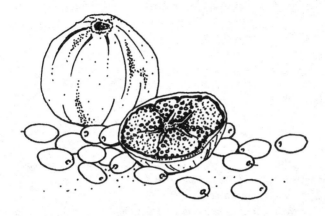

Italian bread, he thought up a hundred different meal ideas based on the principles of the Hay diet. The result was astonishing for him; in two years, he'd lost the extra two stone and had rid himself of the avascular necrosis.

GLUCOSE – BODY FUEL

While the Hay diet has worked for a number of people, it's probably too much of a jump from our normal eating habits for most of us to take very seriously. A low-fat, high-carbohydrate diet will help to keep most major illnesses at arm's length, while fibre alone can work its own miracles. Fibre delays the energy or glucose being absorbed, which is good news in particular for diabetics; this controls the demands placed on the pancreas which is responsible for the production of insulin. Glucose is possibly the most important fuel for the body. It is carried around the body in the blood, and cells which need it absorb it on its way. It's vital that our glucose levels remain pretty stable all the time; if they don't, the brain, which is particularly sensitive to a change in level, will respond by sending messages to the rest of the body. If your glucose levels plummet because you haven't been eating enough fibre to regulate the flow, you'll become irrational and confused, tired or aggressive, and too much of a drop can even make some people faint. Munching into a chocolate bar or drinking something sweet will send the levels shooting up, giving you a temporary high, but confusing your brain and body even more.

The body has its own defence system against our erratic eating habits. It can cope with the fact that, for example, we might be constantly side-tracked by particularly persuasive advertisements, producing its own hormones to keep our glucose levels fairly stable. Insulin is one of them and comes into play when our glucose levels are too high by taking the glucose out of the system and putting it into store for a while. In diabetics, too little insulin is produced and they have to compensate by injecting it into the bloodstream.

Insulin is generally found in higher levels in people who are very overweight and creates a vicious circle: it tends to encourage the body to deposit rather than burn up fat. Changing to a low-fat, high-fibre diet and getting more exercise will give you an opportunity to break the cycle and start losing the excess weight.

THE BOTTOM LINE

Just before it leaves the body fibre has a major job to do in the colon, the area in which some of the biggest killers, including bowel cancer, can grow. The colon is the epicentre of the body's activity; it's like a huge recycling plant, hiving off hormones to be reabsorbed into the blood supply and binning the host of potential carcinogens which attempt to interfere with cells. The arrival of the fibre in the colon vacuums up the waste which the body doesn't need, and is possibly the most important part of the digestive process. More diseases grow in the colon than anywhere else in the body and it is essential to keep it clean. Undigested fibre such as wheatbran encourages beneficial bacteria to grow, which results in the faeces becoming larger and softer and therefore more easily passed out.

Ideally, the process of emptying out waste matter should not be something we worry about too much, unless we fail to oil the wheels with enough regular fibre. Constipation, as well as a long list of very nasty diseases, could be the end result of a defective system but is easily remedied by a good breakfast and a regular supply of fruit and vegetables. Fibre is one of the easiest items to include in a diet of real foods, and one which can make a very real difference to your life not just for now but, more importantly, for your long-term health.

EATING ENOUGH FIBRE

- Eat breakfast and choose wholegrain cereal.

- Eat wholemeal bread, pasta, brown rice and barley.

- Fruit is full of fibre; eat as much as you like.

- The skin of the fruit is where the fibre lies; don't peel your apples and pears.

- Pulses are packed with fibre; add them to soups, casseroles, curries, etc.

- Use wholemeal flour in baking.

TWO

THE F FACTOR

Everyone knows that a good diet is essential for long-term health; part of the reason that most of us can't be bothered is probably because it feels like an insurance policy – something to put off until . . . well, later. But if we could find a diet which would make us look better in a matter of weeks, give us energy and make us feel more lively, then we'd like to know about it. Funnily enough, there *is* something which does all that – and more. It's called fibre and it's the key ingredient in your new approach to life.

We're slowly coming to grips with the theory that what we put into our bodies is linked to the way we look and feel. We've got more information about food and health at our fingertips, there are more adverts on TV which give simple advice on getting the best from our bodies, and there's plenty of great food available all year round to ensure that we get what we need. The best food needn't be expensive, with fruit, vegetables and cereals coming high on the list of nutritionists' best buys.

Judging by the food advertisements on TV, Britain seems to be gripped by an obsession with healthy eating. We've got a vast choice of breakfast cereals, lean lunches and cholesterol-lowering spreads which guarantee us – according to the ads – a fun-filled, action-packed life. You'd think that the British would have more energy, be more sporty and have better bodies than just about anybody else on the beach. We should be posing with the best of the Scandinavian beauties but instead our spotty skins, greasy hair, cellulite and lethargy have become national symbols of our couch-potato lifestyles.

Illness is the last bid for the body to send urgent messages to the brain to *do* something. Most of us in the Western world are now so out of touch with our bodies that those messages can reach us too late, but we can learn to look for earlier signals that something is about to go badly wrong. Skin, hair, eyes and energy levels are dead give-aways. If your eyes aren't clear, your hair is dull and you feel tired all the time, it might be an idea to look at what you're eating. Your looks reflect what is going on inside your body and, as more people begin to recognise the signs, it's going to become embarrassing to be such a walking advertisement for a bad diet.

It could be only a matter of time before people start to notice that you're constipated or suffering from piles. It might be difficult to fight the urge to lean across and gently ask the red-faced, sweating diner on the next table if he's heard of olive oil. His cholesterol level could almost be engraved on his forehead, so close is he to a heart attack. The varicose veins which stare angrily from the legs of some middle-aged women are a testament to bad circulation, and in some cases are easily cured but are generally ignored. A bowl of wheatbran-based breakfast cereal every day could change those women's lives. The 16-year-old schoolgirl, longing to be as glamorous as her newly svelte friends whose waistlines seem to have taken a deep breath in as their breasts filled out, broadcasts her despair via an eruption of spots. She probably takes solace in a chocolate bar, but if only she knew she'd radiate vitality if she had a good breakfast and plenty of fruit and vegetables throughout the day.

More worryingly, one in five people die in this country of diet-related diseases, and the figures are just not dropping. Half the adult population is overweight, and heart disease and

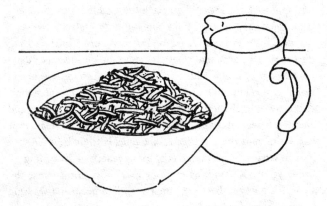

cancer are at epidemic proportions even though we are beginning to catch on to the fact that fibre, olive oil, red wine and lots
of fruit and vegetables could reverse this in a very short time.
The other half of the population is similarly obsessed by food,
with 60% of women at any one time confessing to being on a
diet. But most of them are wasting their time – a low calorie
intake actually slows the metabolism, making it much harder to
burn off any fat. They're on to a loser from the outset. Fatties
and thinnies alike are running the same risk of disease according to latest studies, ramming home the nutritionist's message –
a low-fat, high-fibre diet is the ONLY way to eat healthily.

YO-YO DIETING

The diet industry has no doubt been hoping that the recent
reports which show that yo-yo eating – the cycle of crash
dieting followed by weight gain – is dangerous would prove to
be unfounded. But recent work has shown that people who
submit their bodies to a constant cycle of weight loss and
weight gain have an increased risk of heart disease. And if that

doesn't make you start to think about the price you'll pay for the temporary loss of your bulges, perhaps the horrifying details will . . .

In 1991, the Department of Health issued a warning on the use of very low calorie diets (VLCDs) by the obese, reporting that this leads to the depletion of essential proteins. Under the conditions of these very debilitating weight-loss programmes in which only 400–600 calories are consumed during the course of the day, the body's basic functions can be impaired, sometimes fatally.

The Department drew particular attention to the liquid diets which have become so popular. Manufacturers of the products had to submit their consumer profile to the Department of Health, and their figures showed that one quarter of consumers were using them for more than the 3–4 week recommended period. The Department's report also said that although some of these diets were associated with an increased risk of mortality, by contrast complete fasting under close supervision for as many as 3–4 weeks carries no such risk. The reason for this apparent anomaly comes down to the amino acid composition of the liquid diets. As most of us haven't a clue about such things, the message is simple – stay away from them; we don't understand enough about the way our bodies work to play around with these kinds of diets. It's much simpler and healthier for mind and body to eat – but eat the right foods.

How many of us, for example, know that very low calorie diets – in liquid or food form – will release large quantities of fat from the tissue, but that only part of this can be burnt up as energy? We know that we often feel sick on these diets, but what we probably don't know is that this is because the rest of the released fat is deposited in the bloodstream, causing nausea.

The liquid diets on the market in this country are generally around 400 calories, and, according to government advice, are

NOT safe for pregnant or breast-feeding women, children or infants, the elderly, and people with a heart condition, diabetes or high blood pressure. It recommends that *everyone* should consult their doctor and think very carefully before starting these diets.

Television programmes like *Watchdog* and *Dispatches* have highlighted the problem and talked to people whose lives have been devastated by yo-yo dieting. Terry Pascoe was Weight Watcher of the year in 1980, shedding 10 stone in less than a year. His success was toasted by slimmers all over the country, and he felt fantastic. His weight loss made him seem important to other slimmers, his photo was in magazines, he looked attractive and he felt that his life had finally turned around. Thirteen years later he's back to 21 stone and feels like a total failure. His story is not unusual; two major diet product manufacturers, who boast stories of stunning weight loss in their brochures, refused to allow *Watchdog* access to their files, which probably give a more realistic picture of their products' success rate. Not surprising, said *Watchdog*, considering that a recent study showed that two thirds of dieters put all the weight back on again within a year.

Apart from the physical dangers involved in very low calorie dieting, your mental health might also be at risk. Depriving yourself of real foods on a liquid diet will be traumatic enough for a body which was built to chew but even more of a problem with the dramatic reduction of real foods is the risk of denying yourself essential minerals and vitamins. Scientists are sure that having such a bad attitude towards yourself is also going to have repercussions on your physical and mental health. A loss of essential vitamins like B1 (found in wheatgerm and whole-grain cereals, bread, meat and nuts), B12 (found in lean meat, liver, kidney, milk, fish and shellfish) and folate (found in offal, lightly cooked greens, fortified breakfast cereals, bananas, citrus fruits and nuts) could contribute to what they call 'psychiatric disturbance'. Of course, this can range from getting a bit ratty to deep depression depending on your circumstances, but in a 1992 study, people who were eating more fruit, cereals and vegetables in a weight-loss diet were found to be much better balanced individuals with higher self-esteem.

THE SWANSEA STUDY

The Swansea study into the relationship between diet and mental health took a random sample of people from the electoral register to test the theory that it was these vitamins and minerals in particular (B1, B12 and folate) that engendered a feeling of well-being. They knew that previous tests had shown a better hand to eye co-ordination, memory and increased intelligence in people eating enough B1 and B12 from a regular diet of fruit, cereals and vegetables. As revealed in Chapter 3, levels of concentration and alertness are much higher in people who eat breakfast; and while nobody – unless they write for the tabloids – is going to get away with the assertion that breakfast cereals make you brainy, it does make sense to feed the brain before making it go to work. You might think that your hips need to lose some weight, but your brain will suffer first.

Questionnaires were sent to 1,000 people in Swansea over the age of 18, asking them to list the foods and drinks they generally ate and drank and to give some idea of how frequently this might be. They were asked to pick from a list including red meat, poultry, tinned and fresh fish, beans, peas, pasta, pies, tarts, eggs, dairy products – all kinds of foods you'd expect to find in the average larder. They were also asked about their health, but in a format which was designed to test for any psychiatric disorders.

Interestingly, the study concluded that it was mainly women – rather than men – whose mental attitude improved with more

B1 and B12. Women were found to be *significantly* more anxious if they failed to eat enough fruit and vegetables in their average diet while men didn't seem to suffer these mood swings – whatever they were eating. This probably comes down to the fact that most men use up more energy than women, and consequently have to eat more. By eating more of a wider range of foods, often unwittingly they manage to keep their vitamins and minerals topped up. For example, menstruating women tend to be deficient in iron, but most men aren't. That doesn't mean that active men seek out foods high in iron, but they'll crave meat – or if they're vegetarian, pulses – for *energy*, without even being aware that these are 'iron foods'. They'll eat bread because they're hungry, and spinach because they want to, not because of any fixation with Popeye-style muscles. This will also apply to women who take a lot of exercise. Active men and women also tend to have less of a problem with self-esteem for a myriad of reasons, and it would take another book to explain even half of them.

On the whole, men don't generally feel the same pressure to be a certain shape and are therefore less likely to deprive themselves of food to lose weight. Even though women tend to know more about nutrition, if a couple undertake to go on a diet together, it's generally the man who loses the weight and keeps it off, and the woman who gets depressed about her comparative failure and sulks with a chocolate bar.

In the Swansea study, women with higher self-esteem were more likely to lose any excess weight through a diet of fruit, cereals and vegetables, while those who were on an endless cycle of depressing weight loss and gain were more likely to go for those liquid diets. People who ate natural foods were also more likely to take more exercise, not from any health kick but simply because it made them feel good. It confirmed what psychologists have known all along – that dieting is firmly linked to low self-esteem and that the soul needs real food just as much as the body.

But it's by no means the end of the world for the food masochist. The study showed that a simple shift to low-fat, high-fibre foods would not only help those hellbent on deprivation to lose weight for good, but would immediately boost their vitamin and mineral intake. Encouraging those liquid dieters to *eat* to lose weight in itself would have cheered them up, but the study also showed that the welcoming back of B1 and B12 into their diet quickly made them look and feel better. If someone in your house decides to give up the packet diets and loses weight on a low-fat, high-fibre diet instead, hold on to your hats – the euphoria might be catching . . .

This kind of diet *will* shift the weight for the vast majority, regulating metabolisms and curing hunger cravings. There's now overwhelming evidence that very low calorie diets can also bring on mild depression too. The fact that successful weight loss by eating a low-fat, high-fibre diet can be accompanied by an elevation of mood should clinch it: dieting is history.

All these findings have opened our eyes to the fact that we really are what we eat. In the more sober nineties we want to know how to live and eat well, lose weight if we've over-indulged or have a weight problem. We've been confused by conflicting advice about food and the way our bodies work and now we demand simple, clear information which will help us to lose weight, look and feel better and prevent disease in later life. Food has been the enemy for too long, seen as nothing more than calories at war with our waistline, and it's time to learn how to enjoy it again. All that punishment does the self-esteem no good at all. A new healthy-eating plan packed with goodness and lots of great food will give you a *much* healthier attitude towards yourself.

For most people, this is a liberation. But while it may be much better for body and soul to kick the seven-day plans out of the window, it can be too much of a freefall for many people who need an imposed discipline to their diet. The fear of taking control of their own food is what drives millions of slimmers to the milk-shake diets in the first place. A plan of low-fat, high-fibre foods regulated to specific times of the day can encourage the more obsessed slimmer to start feeding themselves again. Susie Orbach, psychologist and author of *Fat is a Feminist Issue*, says that this is a crucial breakthrough. 'Dieting is one of the most common ways of feeding low self-esteem because you're depriving yourself of something you really need,' she explained. Eating disorders are a tremendously complicated issue from which many women – and not just those diagnosed as anorexics and bulimics – suffer.

EATING DISORDERS

Karen is an anorexic who has only just turned the corner and started to eat three meals a day. She explained how much of a weapon against the world starving yourself can be. 'If you have an enormous amount of anger to throw against the world which has caused you so much misery – whatever that is – starving can be the most effective way of cutting yourself off from it. It gives you a great deal of control and, because it's generally a big secret which only you know about, you feel very powerful.' Believing that fibre will help to lose and regulate weight is difficult for people with eating disorders. 'Most of us have a very old-fashioned approach to losing weight: oils and carbohydrates are the horror foods, and telling us to eat potatoes and pasta is like asking us to cut our heads off. These days I do eat pasta or some other carbohydrates for lunch,' says Karen, 'but even though I feel much better for the rest of the day because I don't feel tired or sick, I still have to live with the guilt of losing my most potent weapon against myself.'

One of the biggest turning points, according to both Karen and Susie Orbach, is when you begin to respect the way your body works. 'The moment you realise that your body is not going to give up on you despite the abuse you're giving it and that, above all, it's trustworthy, then you'll begin to have more respect for it and therefore yourself,' explains Orbach. She suggests taking some time to listen to what your body needs. 'If it's crying out for cheesecake – eat cheesecake for as long as it takes your body to say whoa, I don't need this. When it does, the thought of eating a slice of cheesecake in the future isn't going to mean that you'll never eat anything else again, which is one of the most terrifying things for people with eating disorders.' Good advice, agrees Karen, but in reality the risk might just be too big for an anorexic. Anorexics should take that risk, says Orbach. 'If they do and they see that they're still in control, then they're over the worst. The long-term effect will be that they'll understand that their bodies aren't the enemy. It might take a long time to get over the psychological problems which started this pattern in the first place, but eating will make them feel better physically, which is a good start when you're dealing with self-hatred.

Orbach spends a great deal of time with women who have eating disorders, and swears that it's not ignorance about food that's the problem. On the contrary, they know more about nutrition than most people because they've followed just about every diet ever published. But as each diet failed and they put the weight back on through bingeing, their self-esteem plummeted even further until the battle was being waged with the psyche rather than the waistline. 'You have to empathise with them,' she said. 'You have to encourage them to take the risk with themselves, and start eating again. If they're eating a low-fat, high-fibre diet, they're going to be eating what they need to become healthy, and the rest – even if it takes a while – will naturally follow.' By learning to make low-fat, high-fibre foods into something to feed your friends and family, the bars around food should gently begin to bend and you'll find a way out of that isolated world you've been living in for so long.

THE FIBRE FOR LIFE DIET

If you feel that it's too much of a leap to adopt a free-form, non-calorie-counting diet, Kellogg's Fibre for Life diet might provide the bridge. It aims to shift one to two pounds per week – the target set by most doctors – and to keep it off. A combination of breakfast, a light meal, a main meal, a dessert and a snack every day would come to between 1,200–1,400 calories for women and 1,500–1,800 for men. Three to four pieces of fruit a day are recommended, and dieters can eat any amount of fruit and vegetables or salad. Some recipes from the diet are listed at the back of this book, along with many other low-fat, high-fibre recipes.

The Fibre for Life diet reinforces all the principles outlined in this book, advising those on the diet to be positive and not to give themselves a hard time if they break the regime once in a while, understanding that this could lead to a sulky binge. It strongly recommends not skipping any meals, especially break-fast, only getting on the scales once a week at approximately the same time of the day, and keeping a progress record. Regular exercise not only helps weight loss but tones up muscles, leaving a slimmer, firmer body. The diet recommends an aerobic exercise like walking, swimming or cycling for 30 minutes at least four times a week. Alcohol should be limited on the Fibre for Life diet, and it suggests a spritzer – half white wine, half mineral water – as a good half-way measure.

The diet is based on the high-fibre content of All-Bran and works on the principle that you'll never feel hungry if you stock up on fibre. As high-fibre foods tend to be low in fat, fill you up and don't stay in your body too long, you won't feel light-headed or deprived. If you take your fibre from carbohydrates, like potatoes, pasta and rice, which are easily burnt off, you will be able to get on with your day while your body gets on with ridding itself of excess weight. All this means an important contribution to keeping your weight stable or losing any excess. More importantly, a proper fibre intake will keep the body so well tuned that a number of serious diseases will be kept at bay (see p. 116ff.).

BURNING OFF THE FAT

Fibre provides energy from the carbohydrates, proteins and fats in which it's stored, but doesn't actually have any calories in itself. The foods in which it's found – potatoes, bread, pasta, and proteins like nuts and pulses, all have calorific value, so don't think that you can eat a sackful of potatoes and expect to get into your jeans for a while. A normal helping of carbo-hydrates and proteins can be easily burnt up, so you won't set about expanding your waistline if you make sure you get enough exercise. By eating more carbohydrates, you won't need to fill up on the fats which are more difficult to burn off and you won't get fat. It's as simple as that.

What about the idea that pasta and potatoes are fattening? This was one of the dieting myths put about in the sixties when the working of the body wasn't as well understood as it is these days. The truth is wonderfully straightforward. Fats are fatten-ing, carbohydrates are fuel, and protein is for muscle. All have a crucial role to play in the repair and growth of the body – otherwise they wouldn't exist in nature's larder – but under-stand their functions and you'll never count a calorie again.

A study in 1991 by French researcher Dr Rigaud confirmed that extra fibre in a reduced-calorie diet packed with fruit, vegetables, cereals, pasta and wholemeal bread could have an effect on weight loss. Overweight subjects who had added 7g of fibre a day to a diet which was 25% lower in calories than normal lost twice as much weight as subjects whose identical diet was supplemented with a non-fibre placebo. The successful group reported that they hadn't felt hungry during the study, while those taking the placebo suffered hunger pangs throughout. Dr Rigaud and his team concluded that the extra fibre slows down the stomach's absorption of nutrients like carbohydrates, proteins and fats. Increasing the excretion of any superfluous remainder meant that there was very little chance of them sitting on the hips.

So put away your diet packs and start living in the real world. Your body is perfectly able to find its own weight level, to rid itself of what it doesn't need, and to make itself glow with inner health. Why not allow 'diet' to mean what it *used* to mean: an eating plan which has nothing to do with deprivation or weight loss?

THE DEATH OF THE DIET

The most successful slimmers are the ones who have given up dieting for life. Health and beauty editor Grace Hill used to be obsessed with getting down to a size 12. She was a big size 14 and very conscious of her body image throughout her twenties. 'I knew the calorific content of every single food item you could think of,' she said, 'and it was like an albatross around my neck. I would lose the weight and feel great, then go out and celebrate and put it all back on again. I was trapped by worrying about how I looked. So I decided to give it all up, eat sensibly and take lots of exercise.' Callanetics changed her body shape by gently toning the inner muscles. 'Now I eat what I want and feel fantastic.' Needless to say, the minute she gave up counting the calories, the weight fell off.

'Depression makes you fat,' explained Carole Ann Rice, fashion and lifestyle editor at the *Birmingham Post*. 'I was fine as a child but got fat in my teens with all the pressures of being a spotty pubescent girl. I started dieting and lost some of it but, when I was in my twenties, I discovered that comfort eating could help me through a trauma, and very soon I was up to twelve and a half stone. The more I ate, the more I hated myself. My self-esteem was rock bottom when a compliment from a total stranger made me feel like a human being again and slowly I began to stop abusing my body. Now I eat anything I want and can wear anything I want.'

Robert Farago, author of *Hypno-Health*, agrees that as soon as you stop giving yourself a hard time about your weight and your inability to stick to diets, you'll lose those extra pounds. 'I've seen people who have been through the mill with dieting and weight gain; some of them have been on forty or fifty diets and probably know more about food than I do. The reason they don't work is because eating badly is a subconscious habit and whatever's happening down there is going to win over any decision on the conscious level.' The answer, he claims, is to stop beating yourself up. 'If it worked, I'd say "hey, it's a great way to lose weight" but it isn't, so don't. I'm not saying don't give yourself a hard time because you're a beautiful person or because God loves you – I'm telling you because it just doesn't work.'

He agrees that diet plans are a bad idea for the person who's hellbent on losing the weight war. 'On day four, they don't eat their 4 oz of broccoli and convince themselves that they're a failure. Who needs that kind of pressure? There's such a wide variety of food out there, why should they stick to a few lettuce leaves and a carrot for lunch?' His patients seemed to have an uncanny habit of craving what they thought was comfort food at around 11 in the morning and 4 in the afternoon. The fact that that comfort food generally seemed to be chocolate was making them fat, until Farago measured their blood sugar levels at these times of the day and explained the results. At mid morning and mid afternoon, their blood sugar or glucose levels had dropped so low that they felt they needed a vital injection of something sweet to send their levels shooting up. This pattern of eating meant that their energy levels were peaking and dropping all day, making their bodies crave food while their subconsciouses were confirming that they really were losers. 'These people were like camels crossing the desert,' said Farago, 'going without breakfast, eating only tiny amounts at lunchtime, and then gorging at night. What did they think was going to give them energy during the day? Did they imagine that energy came from the Fourth Dimension?' Farago explains to his patients that in order to be healthy they *need* that energy, and that in order to stop giving themselves such a hard time on the subconscious level they have to start feeding themselves with wonderful delicious foods.

THINKING THIN

As we wrestle with the fact that many of our problems could all be in the mind, and that therefore it really is up to us to do something about it, we're beginning to look around at the evidence. It's no coincidence that overweight people tend to eat more quickly and in larger quantities than thin people. Food for the naturally slim person means eating when they're hungry, and stopping when they've had enough. Look at the way your friends eat; do the thin people tend to leave food on their plates? Do the overweight people eat their food like they're starving, and virtually lick the plate clean? Thin people listen to their bodies; there's no mental dilemma about whether to have another helping or not – if they feel they can fit it in, they will; if they don't, they won't. It's simply not a big deal.

If you're unhappy with your eating habits, eating better food that has an almost immediate effect on your body – making you more energetic, alert and look better – is a great kick-start. But the way we eat comes from deeply established habits, so don't give yourself a hard time if you can't slow down your eating at first. Eating quickly might have started in the race at school mealtimes or in the bosom of a large family where survival of the fittest meant gobbling down your food so you could be first in line for seconds. Fibre takes care of a lot of this. You have to chew it a lot more than fatty foods which slip down your throat, so adding more bread and 'big' vegetables like greens is going to make it much more difficult to gulp your food down.

BODY WORKS

So how does it all work then? It's easy to read the testimony of successful slimmers, but how can you make it work for you? Knowing what your body does with the food and exercise you've been told to give it will go some way to stopping the endless cycle of pollution, punishment and pig-out which has left it in such a state.

First of all, the main thing to remember is that your body *needs* food and you should never have to feel guilty about eating fresh foods like fruit and vegetables. White meat, like chicken, is fine as long as it's lean and not covered in fatty skin. Occasional red meat is OK too, if it's not surrounded by a wedge of fat. Secondly, the principle of losing weight is *always* the same – eat fewer of the calories found in fat, eat more fibre, and burn off anything your body doesn't need through regular exercise. Everyone wants to know the secret of successful weight loss, yet if you look beyond the titles of the Bikini, Hip and Thigh and F-Plan diets, the message is always the same – cut down the fat, eat more fibre and watch the pounds drop off and stay off. Understanding that the body needs so much more than a trimmer waistline will hopefully help you to put your weight dilemma in context.

DIGESTION

It might help to think of the body as a factory where every organ, hormone and nutrient has a job to do, interacting with each other when they need to and keeping a respectful distance when they don't. When food enters the body the conveyor belt of the digestive process bursts into action, which, if you're eating and digesting properly, will hum along perfectly happily right through to 24–36 hours later when it dumps anything it doesn't need in your loo. If it doesn't, something's wrong and you'll know about it.

So let's get technical. The cycle starts with the digestive process. As we chew food, our gastric juices begin to flow. The longer we chew, the more saliva we produce to break up the food and send it on to the next stage. As it gets to the stomach, it's immediately set on by the acids which take off the nutrients they want and break it down again for the next stage. The food is now only semi-digested as it passes into the small intestine where enzymes from the pancreas and bile from the liver break it down even further. By now, that tuna sandwich has become a set of proteins, carbohydrates and fat. Along with their vita-mins and minerals these are then absorbed in their separate units through the intestinal wall into the bloodstream.

Some of the food is not needed, and is carried into the large intestine to make bacteria which service our natural defence system. All during this time, rhythmic contractions of the gut are propelling the waste material from the food through the intestine. If you're drinking your 1–2 litres of water a day, the fibre you've been eating will swell and push through the gut and out of your body smoothly and effortlessly. Cancer experts believe the more quickly the fibre expels the carcinogens present in their benign form in most foods, the better. While it is in the large and small intestine, fibre also disarms the cholesterol and bile salts which are partly responsible for heart disease and gallstones.

Your tuna sandwich with a scraping of polyunsaturated margarine on wholemeal bread and a couple of spinach leaves with a little low-fat mayonnaise is just what the body wanted. It sees it more as protein, carbohydrate and fat containing fibre, calcium, magnesium, potassium, sodium, sulphur, iodine, selenium, and zinc. It's happy that vitamins A, D, E, K, B1, B2, B3, B6, B12, C and folic acid are all being absorbed into the bloodstream, and that you chewed it well enough for your gastric juices to make it all so easily digested.

As long as the glucose levels in the bloodstream remain stable, the body will continue chugging through its process in a calm, reliable way. But erratic eating and a shortfall in the nutrients which come from carbohydrates, proteins and fats will put a spanner in the works, clogging up the waste disposal system and playing havoc with energy levels, appetite, concentration and even causing premenstrual syndrome.

GETTING THE BALANCE RIGHT

A low-fat, high-fibre diet sounds easy enough to get your head around by now, but it all gets a bit confusing when you read that the body needs the right balance of foods and in fairly precise amounts. Quite simply, the kind of foods discussed in *Fibrenetics* will give you everything you need in the way of vitamins and minerals but, as information is the key to better long-term health, it won't hurt to take a closer look at the small-print.

In short, we should be getting a lot of the macro ('big') nutrient group. These are the proteins, fats and carbohydrates which give us the energy we need on a daily basis, and to repair our bodies when they need it. On the other hand, we only need a small amount of micro ('small') nutrients, the vitamins and minerals which have a specific function in digesting the food, helping the nervous system to work properly, and keeping the blood supply healthy. The food we buy in the supermarket contains both macro and micro nutrients.

PROTEINS

We need proteins to grow, maintain and repair our cells. About 17% of the body is formed by protein, including skin, hair, nails, muscle and bone. Have a quick look at your nails and hair. If you've got white spots on your nails, and your hair looks like it needs a holiday, stock up on some poultry, shellfish, eggs, cheese, yoghurt, milk, and pulses such as beans, peas, lentils and nuts.

As a nation, we do well with our protein intake, so no sermon here. However . . . .

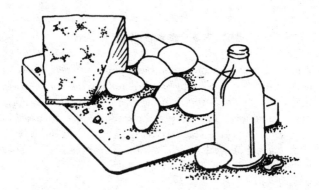

FATS

You may think that you've got your fats sussed just because you buy low-fat yoghurt and 'I Can't Believe It's Not Butter', but the majority of people in the UK still don't understand what fats are all about. Our bodies have no way of telling us immediately if we've been eating too much of the stuff in the same way as they do with carbohydrates. It's difficult to feel full up on fat, and so it's easy to slip it into our diet and not notice until we're a stone heavier.

Energy is stored in the body as both carbohydrate and fat. Carbohydrates are stored in the liver and muscle as glycogen – the long chains of sugar which tide us over until our next meal and give us short bursts of energy. If marathon runners run out of glycogen, their legs will wobble and give way. This store of carbohydrates amounts to very few calories – perhaps 1,000 in the average woman. But *fat* stores are kept in our reserve 'tank' and are supposed to see us through times of famine and hardship. This tank is huge, and the same average woman can store about 125,000 calories of fat in it. Obese people can have something like half a million calories locked away for a rainy day. If they're not burning it up, it'll be sitting on their hips and thighs for a very long time.

Because the tanks are so different in size, an extra few thousand calories slipping into the fat reserve would go unnoticed. But if we suddenly ate another 1,000 calories worth of carbohydrates, we'd burst – or certainly feel as though we were about to. And scientists have recently noticed that while we immediately begin to burn off starches and sugars if we've overfilled our tanks, nothing happens if we eat too much fat. It's as if it slips in unnoticed. The body doesn't seem to compensate at all for this excess fat in the diet, and only tells us where we've gone wrong when it's almost too late and our cholesterol levels and waistlines reach unacceptable figures.

These are important findings for people who want to lose weight. They show that the body is very well designed to cope with the carbohydrates and proteins, but is easily fooled by very high levels of fat. Proof positive that we should give the poor old potato a break, and stop blaming it for weight gain. Fats are the *real* villain of the piece, not only in the weight war but also in the battle against heart disease and cancer.

But not *all* fat is a problem. On the contrary, the fat in olive oil is positively good for us. It will always be high in calories but, eaten in reasonable quantities, fat is a vital part of our diet. We need it for tissue growth and muscle repair, but most of us are buying the wrong kind of fat. There are two kinds: saturated (hard fat like butter, fat on meat, or hard cheese) and unsaturated fat which is the liquid fat we use for cooking. The exceptions are coconut and palm oil which, although liquid, *are* high in saturated fats.

Saturated fats are the ones which can lead to heart disease and some cancers. An excess can raise the amount of cholesterol in the blood causing a blockage in the circulation. This becomes really dangerous when so much cholesterol is in the system that it has to be dumped on the inner walls of the arteries, causing them to fur up and restrict the flow of blood into the heart.

Check out your cholesterol level and whether there's a history of heart disease in your family. People who may not be overweight are still likely to have a high cholesterol level if they're consuming too much saturated fat. The most obvious indication of having high cholesterol is simply being fat, but some people have higher metabolisms than others which burn off a lot of the body fat, and make them thinner while still having a high cholesterol level. If you're a middle-aged man, eating too much butter, cream, and fat on your meat, get yourself an appointment with your doctor as soon as possible – you're bang in the middle of the high-risk category. The

Coronary Prevention Group put 5.2 as a desirable level to aim for, and 5.8 as about average in this country. Anything higher than 6 could be a potential problem, and 8s and 9s are a sure sign that you're well on the way to heart problems in middle age. Cholesterol tests should be carried out in the right medical environment. There's no point in knowing that you're 8.4 if you haven't a clue what that means and what to do about it. And you may need immediate treatment.

The good news about fats is that a whole new concept of eating in this country has emerged from the news that we should be eating more monounsaturated fat – in other words, olive oil. As mentioned earlier, studies have shown that one of the best diets in the world is found in the Mediterranean where fresh fruit and vegetables, cereals, olive oil, red wine and very little meat are responsible for the lowest records of heart disease and diet-related cancers in the world. Using reasonable amounts of olive oil instead of butter in cooking is not going to tear you away from your low-fat, high-fibre habit either – remember we do need *some* fat, and the kind of foods you'll be serving it with are more likely to be fibre-packed pasta and vegetables. You're not very likely to pour it over your pre-packed chicken biryani or your beefburgers and chips, are you?

It's not just heart disease which is held to ransom by the cholesterol-reducing properties of olive oil. The anti-oxidants in olive oil act as a kind of detergent on the cholesterol, making sure that it doesn't clog the arteries. From the breast to the bowel, this little army of anti-oxidants puts up barriers to prevent cancer-causing free radicals attacking the body's cells and causing havoc by disrupting their normal multiplication. The first sign of cancer is abnormal cell reproduction.

Cutting down on fats is easy enough. Cut off the extra fat on meat, go for white meat rather than fatty beef or lamb, and eat more fish and vegetables. Yoghurt and fromage frais are better than double cream, and just as versatile.

FAT FILE

Fromage frais		Yoghurt		Cream	
Plain*	7% fat	Greek	7.5% fat	Single	19.1% fat
Fruit*	5.8%	Plain	1.5%	Whipping	40%
Very low fat*	0.2%	Low fat	0.8%	Double	48%

*Roughly half the fat is saturated

Crème fraîche
This is a cream product imported from France and has roughly the same fat content as double cream.

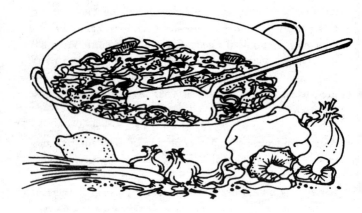

Stir frying in a small amount of liquid fat such as olive oil is better not only for the heart, but also for the waistline; whisking the food around a wok means that the fat barely has time to touch the sides of the food, let alone seep inside. Stir frying vegetables which are served in an almost raw state also means more vitamins are left intact.

CARBOHYDRATES

Gradually we're understanding that pasta and rice are not going to make us put on weight – unless, of course, we eat huge amounts of them and sit watching TV all day. Starch is a carbohydrate in which plants store food, and, as any athlete will tell you, is the main source of energy for the body. We eat that starch in potatoes, pasta and rice, and convert it into glycogen which is then stored until we need some energy. It is then dutifully pulled out of its store, turned into glucose, and suddenly we've got enough energy to do the things we want to do. A plate of pasta is nothing more daunting than a tasty fuel to burn off.

Without carbohydrates in the diet, the body has to get its energy from other 'tanks' – the reserve stores which are not designed to be drawn from and which might not be able to provide enough, or the right kind of energy. Taking energy from muscle tissue, for example, will issue a sharp warning from the muscle – a burning sensation telling you to lay off – to get your energy from somewhere else because it needs it to repair itself and grow. Remember that the heart is the most important muscle in your body and if you start using its resources, it's not going to like it.

Dr Victor Cross, founder of Medicine for Dance and the medical adviser for the Birmingham Royal Ballet, explains that fibre-packed carbohydrates are absolutely vital for dancers. 'Dancers are unique among athletes because they have to maintain a very low body fat. An average slim woman has about 20% body fat and someone who's a bit chubby has 30%

but a female dancer has between 10–12%. She has to eat energy foods to keep her going all day, and that means that she has to eat a lot of carbohydrates which won't make her fat – like pasta and cereals. You have to make the distinction between good and bad carbohydrate sources,' warns Cross. 'Chocolate cake is also a source of carbohydrate . . . ' Dr Cross advises his dancers to eat 60% carbohydrates, 20% fat and 20% protein. The fat can come from meat even without its visible fat cut off, or even a teaspoon of mayonnaise.

All athletes have to load their muscles with glycogen – the energy which comes from carbohydrates – but the difference between dancers and other athletes is that dancers have to use it immediately while athletes can store it up before a race or a fight. 'Dancers work eight-hour days,' explained Dr Cross, 'and need their energy for afternoon rehearsals as well as an evening performance. That means they have to eat well every single day.' If they don't, they're in trouble. In 1989 a study of classical ballet dancers showed that 32% of all injuries on stage happened during the evening when energy levels were low. 'This had nothing to do with stage fright,' said Dr Cross, 'their muscle state just wasn't up to scratch, and that's because they probably hadn't eaten properly the day before.' A good diet for a dancer would always include a high-quality cereal for breakfast – Dr Cross recommends Fruit 'n Fibre – a light snack of fruit and an orange juice for lunch, followed by a proper meal at teatime packed with fibre-filled carbohydrates like brown rice, baked beans on toast, a baked potato or pasta.

Ballet dancers have to eat at teatime, which isn't ideal, but it's the only option with their schedule. Dr Cross insists that they must have some source of energy at midday if they're to make it through the day. 'Those adverts for glucose drinks are quite misleading,' he said. 'You wouldn't actually catch a top athlete drinking one of those before a race. I told my dancers to try a pint of orange juice or a banana before going back into rehearsals, and when they did they said that they were amazed to find that they didn't feel tired by the end of the day.' That's because they need to load up the muscles with energy from carbohydrates which the muscle can then store as glycogen.

Boxers and athletes have a different routine which allows them to rest for a couple of days before a fight or a race. 'It's just like recharging a battery,' explains Dr Cross. 'They'll pack in the pasta and then sit around for two days, making sure that they don't train or use any great amount of energy before their big day.' The fact that they make sure that sex is off the menu for that period is a testament to how seriously they take their regime.

Most female dancers, in spite of the fact that they expend much more energy than most other women, only need 1,000 calories a day because their bodies have been programmed since they were very young to work on such a small intake. This, according to Dr Cross, makes a nonsense of calorie-controlled diets. 'If a dancer needs to lose weight she has to burn it off through aerobic exercise. Normally ballet is a series of stops and starts, so they don't burn as much off as you'd think but they will need their energy for prolonged sessions throughout the day. The only way for anyone to lose weight and maintain it is by eating properly and increasing their exercise.'

Exercise	Calories burnt off per hour
Fast walking	300
Jogging	350
Aerobics	500
Step aerobics	600

If you walk a reasonable distance most days, ride a bike, swim or play sport regularly – or even if you're particularly active in the bedroom – you'll find that carbohydrates will never make you fat; on the contrary, they'll give you the energy you need to do your chosen activities well.

SUGAR

The body breaks sugar and starch from carbohydrates down into glucose which we need for energy. We never *need* to add sucrose (table sugar) to our food – we only eat it because we like it. We've always treated ourselves to sweet things and all over the world people still suck sugar cane as a natural snack. The macho men of the Baka tribe in the Cameroon rain forest still hoist themselves up branchless trees and risk being stung to death to ransack the honeycombs of the beehives, and all because the lady loves sugar. When sugar cane is pressed and its juice is concentrated, its non-sugar components are extracted, leaving pure sucrose for the Western world to enjoy. Even brown sugar, which many people think is better for them than white, is pretty redundant as far as your body is concerned. It might help you to know that the palate is a creature of habit, and it could only take you three days without sugar to forget that chocolate, toffees and biscuits ever existed. The psychological reasons for your binges on biscuits might take a little longer to sort out, but if you give your body a treat by eating more cleansing fibre in fresh fruit, and vegetables roasted and drizzled with a little extra virgin olive oil, you might find it easier to kick the habit than you ever thought possible.

VITAMINS AND MINERALS

Most vitamins were discovered early this century when doctors began to realise the role they could play in curing serious diseases. The B vitamin thiamin was among the first to be recognised in food and was used to cure beri-beri, the cause of a great deal of serious stomach upsets in the last century. As more B vitamins were discovered, experts who had more important things to think about than naming each of them, numbered them from B2 to B15. Seven have since been deemed non-essential so we're left with a classified team of eight.

These micro, or 'small' nutrients, are essential for keeping the body reacting properly. While the nutrients like fibre get on with the job of actually getting us through the day, helping us get energy from our food, making our brains alert and stopping us feeling hungry, vitamins are the engineers, constantly tweaking our internal defence system to make sure that it's all in working order. They all have their job to do *every* day, and don't simply assist in an emergency. Keeping them topped up by eating plenty of fruit, vegetables and cereals means you won't need supplements. Some vitamins in particular have to be topped up more than others. These are the water-soluble types; vitamins B and C fall into this category and have to be regularly replenished as they pass out of the system in urine. Fat-soluble vitamins like A, D, E and K are found in liver, fish oils, egg yolk and greens and can be stored in the liver for days.

Minerals have special jobs to do in the body, maintaining the growth of teeth, hair and bones, before passing out of the body once their job has been done. Like vitamins, they pass through urine, sweat and faeces, and have to be stocked up regularly. If you eat a well-balanced diet you won't need to take supplements.

SALT

Salt is one of the micro nutrients which we need in tiny amounts – something like half a teaspoon a day. It contains essential sodium and chlorine, and we must replace what we lose every day in urine, faeces and sweat. But it is also a potential health hazard if we take too much of it. High blood pressure can lead to strokes, heart disease and kidney failure, which may be due to too much salt in the diet. However, there are also more important factors such as obesity, smoking, alcohol and lack of exercise to be taken into account. Water retention is also the result of excessive salt intake: people with a weight problem might find that they are simply full of water, and cutting out on the salt might mean losing inches quickly and safely.

Try seasoning your food with herbs instead, which have all sorts of curative value according to the ancient herbalists whose methods have been preserved in modern herbal medicine. Garlic, spices, pepper and fruit juices will give your cooking plenty of flavour without any risk to your body.

WATER

The body's need for water becomes a raging thirst if you don't give it enough and you're eating a good quantity of fibre. Fibre is a demanding little thing, needing water to complete its action of sweeping the body, and will make sure that you treat your body properly. Water works hand in hand with fibre to detoxify the system. Fibre absorbs the water which has flushed all the toxins and waste into the colon, and together they form the large soft stools which so effectively expel everything our bodies don't want or need. Water is the most potent dynamic nature could have provided. Bottled or filtered water is probably the best bet, especially if you're travelling abroad, because your immune system won't have programmed itself for the different bacteria at large in the tap water.

There are some general rules about water which most people know but which are worth repeating: don't fill the kettle from

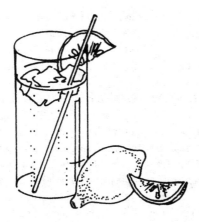

the hot-water tap as it comes from a tank which is being constantly reheated and allowed to cool. This may affect the mineral content, and it could fall again as your kettle boils. Remember to empty the kettle after you've used it too.

Fluoride has been added to much of our national water supply, but if you think that drinking tap water alone will be good for your teeth, think again. You'll get really healthy teeth from regular brushing and, most importantly, eating a good diet rich in calcium from bread, greens, cheese and some milk and raw foods which, if really chewed, build up your fluoride protection through their action with the saliva.

CAFFEINE

It's worth applying that boring old adage 'everything in moderation' to drinking tea and coffee – and don't forget that you'll get a caffeine kick from some colas and chocolate too.

While most people don't get more than a pleasant buzz from caffeine, taken in excess it can produce anxiety attacks, mood swings, the shakes, insomnia, heart palpitations, sweating and weight loss. The wonderfully titled 'restless leg syndrome' is another symptom of caffeine poisoning, and describes the involuntary thrashing around in bed that millions of people either experience themselves or have to put up with from their partner. You'd think that anyone who suffered *any* of these complaints would give up caffeine, but it *is* a drug, and going without can be more painful than addicts think it's worth. If you're addicted, try cutting down over 2–3 weeks. Small amounts of caffeine can actually be beneficial, and help with concentration. Some people just wouldn't be able to get started in the morning without their coffee, and others find it makes a great way to end a meal. To deprive them of such a pleasure is defeating the whole object of mind and body health.

EATING TO LOOK BETTER

Vitamins and minerals are the key to looking great. If you've longed for shining hair, white, sparkling eyes and clear skin, look no further than your supermarket. And it's so easy; have a great fibre-packed breakfast, drink loads of water through the day, eat plenty of fresh fruit and vegetables, and get some exercise. In the simplest foods, you'll find all the vitamins you need, plus minerals like zinc which promotes skin repair; it's also particularly useful for reducing stretch marks during pregnancy.

The very best way to look after your hair is to eat wholemeal cereals, bread, brewer's yeast and liver. They all provide vitamin B complex which will give it a kick start and also reduce the risk of losing your hair. Some nutritionists believe that oily fish keeps hair shiny and glossy. If you suffer from dandruff you might not be getting enough selenium (found in any food grown in soil), zinc or vitamins C and B6 (found in whole-grains, potatoes, bananas, fatty fish, lean meat and greens).

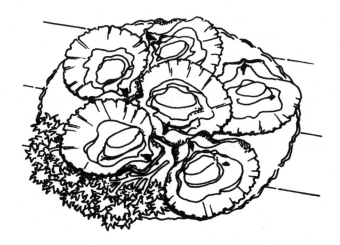

Zinc, found in seafood, cereals and red meat, and calcium from dairy products and dark green leafy greens like spinach, will look after your nails. Eyes will look better if you follow the same rules and make sure you take lots of exercise which will increase the supply of blood and oxygen to them.

SKIN DISORDERS

PSORIASIS

This is undoubtedly one of the most serious skin complaints. It manifests itself in great red welts over the face and body. Although only people with a hereditary disposition to psoriasis will suffer from it, it is exacerbated by stress and if you ignore its symptoms, your body will send further messages such as fatigue, insomnia and stomach ulcers. Psoriasis is a side effect of the body being put on stress alert. Naturopaths believe that it can be neutralised by drinking the juice of a raw potato or, perhaps more palatably, by eating a lot of fatty fish. Mackerel is particularly good. But while eating good food with friends or family should make you feel more relaxed, don't take short cuts and imagine that you can ignore the stressful situation which set off the alarm in the first place. Think about it; there's always a way out of a problem. If you recognise the reason and simply can't do anything about it for now, at least eat and exercise properly in the meantime – it'll help you sleep at night and be more alert during the day to deal with the situation.

BLOCKED PORES

The skin is made up of millions of pores which allow the skin to breathe. They are the end of the tunnel for the trillions of follicles which provide access from the sweat-producing seba-ceous glands to the surface of the skin. But these can get blocked if you don't get enough vitamin A from fatty fish, egg yolk, greens and carrots. In the worst cases it produces very unpleasant-looking knobbly skin all over the body, but particu-larly on the back of the arms and front of the thighs.

ENLARGED FOLLICLES

This is also called dyssebacea or nasolabial seborrhoea, and is characterised by large follicles around the sides of the nose and cheeks. The pores are blocked with a dry, yellow sebaceous substance which flakes off in the way that dandruff does on your scalp. Riboflavin or B2 is the answer, and you'll get it in brewer's yeast, fortified cereals, greens, milk, cheese, meat and fish.

AGEING

Now that we're generally living longer, nutritionists are being encouraged to deal with the dietary needs of a new sub-group – the older middle-aged 50–70-year-olds. Because many people in this group are still working and leading active lives, their needs are different to the more traditional relaxed lifestyle of the elderly. Life expectancy is now about 75 across Europe compared with 47 in Britain at the beginning of the century. In America the over-85s are the fastest-growing segment of the population, and in Britain, many of our own health pioneers are still living proof of their findings. Sir Richard Doll, the man who made the link between cancer and smoking, is still at his desk in Oxford's Peto Institute, filing his studies for the Imperial Cancer Research Fund despite the fact that most people of his age would have retired 20 years ago. Dr Denis Burkitt, the fibre man himself, was delivering lectures across the world up to the time he died early in 1993 aged 82. The architect of the Mediterranean diet told the world 50 years ago that olive oil and red wine can reduce cholesterol levels and prolong life. Professor Ancel Keys is 90, yet only now are his lectures being taken seriously.

These people certainly know not only how to extend their life-span, but how to stay more mentally alert than most of us ever were in the first place. Of course making a major contribution to the understanding of world health would probably give you a reason to live longer, and feeling valued certainly helps to keep one's all-important self-esteem as high as it should be. Good housing, mental stimulation and a happy home life all help to encourage the brain to give the body a better chance.

With the decline of the extended family, and because more people are living longer, more elderly people are living on their own. Consequently there has been a growing awareness of the nutritional problems of the elderly. Experts believe that a better diet could help to slow the withering of bone and body, deterioration of sight and the immune system, and keep the free radicals which hasten this degeneration as well as the onslaught of cancers at bay.

Of course, the better health of such a growing number of people would greatly benefit any country's economy, not least because they are more likely to continue to work. It has been estimated by American experts that even a ten-year delay in the onset of diseases common among the elderly would save several billions of dollars in health care.

B6 is the main vitamin which the elderly should be getting more of in their diet. Between 50% and 90% are getting less than the recommended allowance set down by the Department of Health. That means eating more wholegrains, fatty fish, nuts, potatoes, cereals, bananas, lean meat, avocados, spinach and green beans.

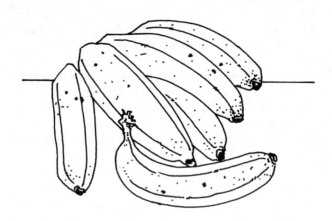

ANTI-OXIDANTS

Every time we breathe in, oxygen gets into our bodies and encourages tiny particles called free radicals to set about destroying our cells. At any age, we automatically counteract this damage with anti-oxidants which are like the body's own home guard. Joining ranks to limit cell destruction by the free radicals, they allow our bodies to regenerate new cells until we start to get old. That's when the home guard begin to need some reinforcements. We make our own anti-oxidants in the body, but need more from food itself to keep the stocks replenished. Eating more foods rich in natural anti-oxidants will boost the ranks and keep the cells regenerating for longer. Dietary anti-oxidants include vitamins A, C, E, beta-carotene, and minerals such as selenium.

In addition to fruit and vegetables, extra virgin olive oil is one of the best sources of anti-oxidants because the less acidic top-of-the-range olives are the ones which are not bruised or split in any way. That means the cells have remained intact, the air and oxygen won't have got to them and their anti-oxidant qualities are in perfect condition to fight off all those free radicals.

Selenium, a mineral from the soil, is found in grains and anything that grows in the ground and is also thought to be a particularly good anti-oxidant.

However, some soils are too rich in selenium, while others have hardly any at all; the ice-age is supposed to have been responsible for some of the depletion of selenium when the water from the melting ice cap leached it along with zinc, iron and calcium from the soil.

The anti-oxidant vitamin E found in egg yolk, wholegrains, greens, vegetable oil and seeds will also protect against the cell damage which actually makes us look old. Our body is programmed to kill off certain cells as we get older so that we literally wind down as we approach death. As our internal body clocks switch off various functions, we stop producing important hormones and our immune system becomes weaker. At the same time the highly active particles or molecules called free radicals are being produced, which then set about reacting with other particles to damage cells and the collagen fibres or elastic tissues in the skin. As they 'cross link', the collagen fibres become tangled, and we begin to look wrinkled as the skin loses its suppleness. This 'cross linking' also causes veins and arteries to harden, limbs to stiffen and muscles to soften.

If this isn't bad enough, lack of exercise and obesity actually speed up the whole process. But nutritionists and naturopaths have been working hard to discover a lifeline, and have concluded that a combination of boosted minerals and vitamins from more natural foods in the diet can have anti-ageing effects. They recommend a low-calorie diet packed with fresh fruit and vegetables with particular emphasis on vitamin E from peanuts, egg yolk, greens, nuts and seeds to slow the ageing of body cells and ward off infection, and a mixture of B vitamins to prevent tiredness and loss of appetite. Bs are found in most foods from wheatgerm and wholemeal cereals to nuts, meats, fish and greens, so it's quite difficult to avoid them.

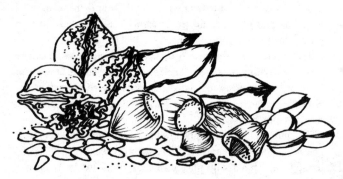

EXERCISE

After eating all this wonderful food, you'll probably find yourself bursting with energy and won't look upon exercise as a chore. In the same way that your body used to scream at you to give it chocolate, it'll now be itching to stretch its legs, climb a mountain, or swim 50 lengths. Well, maybe 20 for now . . . Just as the body needs food, it really does *need* exercise.

Exercise helps to curb hunger, for those who are interested in losing weight. It also slows the process of digestion, and increases the metabolic rate. If you've been used to crash dieting, you might find that your body has become flabbier with each new diet, even though you may actually have lost quite a bit of weight – for a while. This is because when you start cutting down on your food intake the body goes on the defensive, shutting off access to the fat stores to save calories. The muscles weaken and valuable muscle tissue is lost. The more you crash diet, the flabbier you'll become. But by burning off the calories and using up more of the body's store of fat through exercise, you'll be doing exactly the opposite of what you were doing on your crash diet. You'll be toning the muscles, giving yourself a sleeker look and, if you keep it up, you'll maintain your body's natural weight level for life.

Apart from improving your circulation, exercise controls blood pressure, and, in the case of diabetics, can even improve tissue sensitivity to insulin. It's great for stress and even better for your sex life. It'll help your posture, make you more alert at work and at home, and could even open up your social life.

Raising a Lycra-clad limb in front of the video may be a start, but if you join a gym, an aerobics class or go dancing, cycling, or for long Sunday walks, you'll find that your body's getting all the exercise it needs without any sense of effort or hardship at all.

VITAMINS AND MINERALS

Vitamin	Sources	Looks after
A	liver, fatty fish, egg yolk, carrot, whole milk, butter, margarine, greens, cheese	skin repair, immune system
D	sunlight, oily fish, egg yolk	bones, teeth
E	vegetable oil, egg yolk, nuts, seeds, peanuts, polyunsaturated margarine, wholegrains, greens	protection of cells
K	liver, greens	aids blood clotting
B1	wheatgerm and cereals, white flour, brewer's yeast, meat, nuts	nervous system, breaks down carbohydrates to provide energy
B2	brewer's yeast, cheese, yoghurt, meat, egg, greens, fortified cereal	energy, repair of body tissue

B3	liver, lean meat, oily fish, tuna, potatoes, peanuts, fortified cereals, wheatgerm	energy, circulation, nervous system
B5	liver, kidney beans, egg yolk, peanuts, wholegrain cereals	hair and skin, breaks down carbohydrates
B6	liver, wholegrains, nuts, egg yolk, fatty fish, banana, spinach, avocado, lean meat, green beans	nervous system, water retention, skin
B12	lean meat, liver, kidney, milk, fish, shellfish, egg	red blood cells, breaks down fat
folic acid	liver, kidney, raw greens, nuts, citrus fruit, banana	red blood cells, DNA formation
biotin	kidney, liver, egg yolk, yeast	processing of fat and protein
C	citrus fruit, berries, potatoes, sweet peppers, greens	tendons, cartilege, ligaments, protects vitamin E

How much exercise do you really get? Look around you. Your TV probably has a remote, the car outside means that you may not have walked any distance for months, and your record collection may be your pride and joy but probably doesn't inspire you to get up and shake your thing. Dancing on a Saturday night used to be a great laugh, but these days you tend to spend it down the pub. Well, surprise yourself and get out on the town. If you can't dance, do what most other people are doing and stay on one spot flailing your arms around. You'll soon find out how much energy that consumes . . . Your heart will thank you for it.

THREE

BREAKING THE FAST

As the concept of dieting finally kicks the bucket, the news that eating a good breakfast is essential for both good health *and* weight loss has never been so welcome. But it's not just the slimmer who should take note of the benefits of a healthy breakfast. The studies examined in this chapter not only show that people who eat breakfast are more alert, energetic and sociable, but they also paint a sad portrait of the breakfast skipper. Fat, irritable and suffering from low self-esteem, he or she is not likely to be very bright, is probably going to have more accidents in the late morning, and will probably be a smoker and drinker. The breakfast skipper is already on course for a heart attack in middle age, will have upset his or her metabolism at an early age and will therefore be addicted to unsuccessful dieting for life. Is this you? If so, you'd better read on.

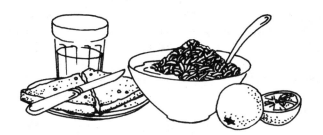

There is hope for the breakfast skipper in the form of a daily bowl of cereal, a slice of toast and a glass of orange juice. It will probably take a leap of faith for the black coffee and cigarette breakfaster to believe that he or she will *lose* weight by eating rather than starving first thing in the morning, but hopefully this chapter will provide the launch pad. Of course, we've always known that eating at the beginning of the day was a sensible thing to do, but who's sensible when they're trying to lose weight? Going without food gives that light-headed feeling people associate with a disappearing waistline. For years, as we tried to squeeze our shapes into somebody else's ideal, we ignored the fact that we couldn't quite concentrate at work, that we'd get unnecessarily ratty with the children, and that our poor partners were spending more and more time at the pub. But those days are over. Food is the answer to losing weight, and no more so than breakfast. Unconvinced? Keep reading.

Many breakfast foods are high in fibre, and all are high in carbohydrate, so it's easy to fill up on low-fat foods which have barely a calorie between them. Cereals like Bran Flakes and All-Bran are delicious with extra fruit which adds to the fibre intake while satisfying the sweeter palate. Once you've had half your daily fibre quota in a couple of mouthfuls, you can rest assured that you'll be getting rid of it within 24–48 hours.

Breakfast eaters have been shown to be generally less likely to gain weight. Even in people who consume the same number of calories over the whole day, those who eat a good breakfast and a lighter evening meal have significantly fewer weight problems than those who concentrate their energy intake later in the day. The message from the nutritionists is simple – eat a lot at the beginning of the day to make sure that you're stocking up on the right nutrients, and you'll spend the rest of the day working it off.

A high-fibre breakfast is more important than just as a means of losing weight effectively. Apart from the essential role it has to play in the prevention of serious diseases like heart disease, cancers and an almost endless list of illnesses of the bowel, nutritionists have now found that a good breakfast is the key to high performance at work and school.

Breakfast means literally that – breaking the fast which might have lasted over 12 hours. Children, who might not have eaten for 16 hours, will be in desperate need of a shot of glucose by the time they get up. Without it, they'll have very little energy for the day ahead, and, while children tend to use up much more than we do when we start to spend most of our days behind a desk, adults can't afford to lose out either.

Studies in Britain, America and Sweden show that missing breakfast can affect behaviour and performance at school and at work, particularly in the late morning. Nutritionists have discovered that including enough fibre in a diet regulates body glucose, and modulates those highs and lows throughout the day. In 1973 a Salford University study looked at the relationship between skipping breakfast and accident rates at a steel foundry. It found that men who hadn't had breakfast were more likely to have accidents in the morning than after lunch, and also before a mid-morning break. When they were then given a drink of glucose for breakfast the accident rate dropped from 34 to 14 per 100 men.

Workers in Swedish factories were also tested on how their performance related to whether or not they were big breakfasters. No surprise that productivity proved to be higher in those workers who had stocked up on their complex carbohydrates and fibre before heading into town. Their colleagues who had skipped their cereal and toast were more likely to be restless and weary by mid-morning and mid-afternoon, as were children, according to a Swedish study on schoolchildren's eating habits. On the days when they'd had a good breakfast, they tended to work faster and make fewer mistakes in subjects like maths which required high levels of concentration. Children who missed breakfast were found to be irritable and unable to concentrate at school. Prolonging the fast can mean low blood sugar and insulin levels which nutritionists now directly relate to poor problem solving – especially by mid morning.

Mothers-to-be also need their fibre for breakfast as constipation is common in pregnancy. Cereals also give them folic acid and iron which are an important part of their diet. But despite the crucial rule a good breakfast plays in our lives, as a nation, we're not eating enough of it. There was a time, as your grandmother will tell you, when the whole family sat down to a plate of bacon and eggs. But have a look at the chart below to see just how much fibre that was giving us compared to the huge amount of fat our bodies really can do without.

BREAKFAST BREAKDOWN

THE GREAT BRITISH BREAKFAST

2 sausages, 1 slice fried white bread,
2 rashers fried bacon, scrambled egg,
1 fried tomato

963 cals, 75g fat, 34g carbohydrate, 1.5g fibre

CEREAL BREAKFAST

1 glass orange juice
1 bowl Bran Flakes with semi-skimmed milk and
1 banana

390 cals, 4.5g fat, 78g carbohydrate, 6.9g fibre

When women started to make up a much larger proportion of the workforce, it became vital to find a less time-consuming option to feed the entire family.

Kellogg's undoubtedly led the way in the breakfast revolution, but the story goes back much further than we might think. Cereals were becoming big business in America in the early part of the century after Dr. Will Kellogg had developed two new health products based on corn and bran. During his experiments in primitive food technology in Michigan he chanced upon a way of flaking cooked wheat to produce a palatable breakfast cereal. But it was his father back in the mid-19th century who began to understand the important effect of fibre on health when he joined the Seventh Day Adventists in Battle Creek, Michigan. John Preston Kellogg's baby daughter had died – unnecessarily, as he thought – and, disgusted at the state of local medicine, he realised that this deeply religious community, dedicated to the health of mind, body and spirit, could offer him what he was looking for for his family. Over the years Battle Creek became known across North America and Europe as a centre for health reform, based on the Adventists' theories of water treatment, diet, rest, exercise and fresh air. The sanatorium began to attract people from all over the world, and Kellogg's son Will was born into the environment of health initiatives which would eventually be responsible for his breakthrough breakfast cereal.

Corn Flakes were the inadvertent result of Will's and his brother's attempts at making a boiled wheat product. They'd run it through the rollers, scraped off the gummy dough with a chisel and were still left with a totally inedible result. When, one weekend, they forgot about a batch of cooked wheat and left it standing until Monday morning, they decided to try to make something of the result. They scraped off the residue and ran it through the rollers to see what happened. The thin flakes of wheat which came out weren't in the slightest bit gummy, and when they tried baking them, they became crisp and vaguely edible. These were developed into Granose Flakes which, tough and tasteless though they were, marked the beginning of flaked cereal technology and were given to the patients at the sanatorium to test. Surprisingly enough, people seemed to go for their health message and within a short time Granose Flakes were selling across America. This inspired Will to try the technique on barley, corn and other cereals, and when rival companies began to make their own wheat flakes, he decided to go all out for what he considered to be the better product. This was the birth of Corn Flakes. The rivals began to go out of business when people realised that – healthy or not – poor quality wheat flakes were not the way they wanted to start their day. Will seized the market, flavoured his Corn Flakes with malt and later sugar, until they became so popular that soon they were even exported abroad.

By 1916, All-Bran had been developed using the same technique of roasting and shredding the cereal, and was taking America by storm. When it arrived in Britain in 1922, the average household was eating eggs, bacon and porridge every morning, and didn't take kindly to going to work on a cold breakfast. The influence of the cereal-eating American public via the new televisions of the fifties and sixties changed our breakfast habits for ever, and now those of us who do eat breakfast – which is still the majority of Britons – tend to start the day with cereal.

Not until nutrition was developed as a science did bran really come back into favour. Even then it suffered an identity crisis, being too closely linked with 'the national loaf', a government gift to the nation during rationing in the Second World War. The British public had never had a bowel movement so good, but bran was still 'war food', and they couldn't wait to get their teeth into the 'real' stuff once again.

But while the trend towards the quicker breakfast of cereal and toast is much better news for the body, many of us are doing without breakfast completely. Young adults are the worst offenders, thinking they haven't got time or that skipping breakfast is the key to losing weight: 14% of people under 55 start the day with no more than a drink, compared to 6% of over-55s, who by that age are probably suffering from the constipation, piles and gallstones a good breakfast would have helped to prevent.

Children eat more breakfast cereals than any other age group: 65% of the toddler to 12-year-old age group will eat a good hearty breakfast on any one day. The carbohydrates in a bowl of cereal mean that they can expend vast amounts of energy without feeling tired, while a child who hasn't refuelled those glycogen stores will be unable to keep up. Studies in Canada have even found that children who go to school hungry are more likely to suffer from low self-esteem and social isolation. Dr Lynn MacIntyre at Dalhousie University found that the hungry child would be apathetic, disinterested and irritable. She explained that he'd be unlikely to be able to concentrate well in class, and consequently would get bored and restless. His energy levels in the playground would be sadly lacking, which means that his schoolmates probably wouldn't have time for him either. MacIntyre reckoned that the more his parents and teachers responded negatively to his behaviour, the more isolated he'd become. Not only is the poor child being ostracised at school, but he's likely to be fat as well. Most breakfast skippers tend to eat more for their evening meal and don't have time to burn it off before bedtime, as the metabolism slows down by the evening. This pattern can lead to early, and often permanent, obesity. Studies show that obese people are much more likely to put weight back on once they've lost it, and tend to go on the kind of very low calorie diets discussed in Chapter Two. This pattern of deprivation once again comes down to low self-esteem which in this case could well have been fostered at school. If Dr MacIntyre's picture of this sad child resembles your son, or daughter – do them a favour, give them some breakfast; they deserve a better start in life . . .

MacIntyre points out that this is not a problem which is exclusive to poorer families; dual-income families can be too busy in the morning to make their children – or themselves – a nutritious breakfast. In most households, the demise of the Great British Fried Breakfast means that the first meal of the day is an easily accessible free-for-all; it's more feasible for a five-year-old to help him or herself to a bowl of cereal than to whip up a quick round of bacon and eggs, and this means that busy parents have no excuse to let anyone leave the house on anything less than a full tank of fibre and carbohydrates.

Blood cholesterol levels were also found to be lower in children who eat breakfast and, in particular, cereals. While higher cholesterol levels are not likely to cause too much trouble in childhood, the build-up could cause serious heart problems later in life. At a stage in life when eating habits are starting to be dictated by body image, it's important to remember that high blood cholesterol caused by skipping breakfast is the result of an upset metabolism. And only healthy metabolisms will free the overweight from a lifetime of dieting.

By the onset of puberty, a vast number of teenagers are starting to skip breakfast, with girls the biggest offenders. Experts report that between 17% and as many as 40% of young people are missing out on the most important meal of the day. As we reach puberty and our bodies go through the most dramatic changes, one of the most important turn-arounds in eating habits can happen. Boys start to eat huge portions of everything as their bodies have a sudden spurt of growth while girls suddenly develop a shape for the first time in their lives. As boys get spotty and gangly, girls tend to become acutely aware of the received opinion of how women should look; it can be with horror that they notice how the sudden appearance of breasts and stomach is not going to make them look like the model Kate Moss. At ten, breasts can be at best a bit embarrassing, at worst a major trauma leading to an eating disorder for life. With puppy fat settling down on hips and stomachs for the next few years, the only option seems to be to start to diet, like everyone else at school. And breakfast is the first casualty. Peer pressure can mean that if you're seen to be eating, then you're not grown up enough to care about your figure. But eating a hearty breakfast at home away from that pressure will not only give teenagers a head start in keeping the weight off and avoiding hunger pangs, it will also maintain a regular metabolism which will keep weight stable throughout life. Studies have also shown that breakfasting teenagers are more likely to know the difference between a healthy snack and a high-fat filler. A much better attitude towards food is fostered in teenagers who understand the relationship between food and energy from the earliest opportunity.

A study which looked at the breakfast habits of 16–17-year-olds who *did* eat in the morning showed that high-fibre cereals were eaten more by middle-class teenagers in the south and east of England. In Scotland and the north, where cereals *were* eaten, they tended to be the pre-sweetened but lower-fibre type like Frosties and Sugar Puffs. The Department of Health recommends that we should be eating 18g of fibre a day, so the Scottish and northern teenagers would have to eat a lot of fruit and vegetables and a good few pieces of wholemeal bread to reach their quota. The availability of fruit and vegetables in Scotland has been severely criticised and is said to explain why the fibre levels there are so poor. The vast distances between some towns in the north means that the hypermarkets aren't as likely to be built in the Highlands as they are in the highly populated commuter belts of the home counties, and distribution to the smaller stores is dictated by customer trends. But, even so, if these under-nourished Scottish and northern teen-agers followed the advice of their grandparents and ate a bowlful of porridge every morning, they'd get an immediate shot of at least 2.1g of fibre.

The teenagers in the study were choosing diets which were leaving them sadly lacking in essential nutrients from zinc to calcium, iron and folates. Young women of child-bearing age should make sure that they're getting enough of all these, but folates in particular will make an important contribution to a healthy baby. Nuts, cooked greens, citrus fruits, bananas, breakfast cereals and liver are where you'll find your folates. The study showed that those eating fortified breakfast cereal without any other major changes to their routine had better intakes of most of the vitamins and minerals. Adding skimmed milk to cereal rather than full-fat milk seemed to make the prospect of a major fibre boost much more attractive to the weight-conscious girls in the group.

This propensity to miss out on essential minerals and vita-mins is one which has serious implications on future health. Studies show that women who skip breakfast are more likely to have 'less appropriate dietary intake patterns' throughout the day, which means they tend not to get enough zinc, copper, calcium and magnesium as well as iron. But men don't seem to fall into the same patterns. Missing breakfast for them tends to be due to lack of time, or to too much stress first thing in the morning, and their eating habits during the day do tend to make up for the lack of nutrients at breakfast.

As the Swansea study in Chapter Two revealed, men don't seem to eat food for health reasons. It tends to be more of a knee-jerk reaction of feeding hunger pangs until, that is, early middle age looms and years of eating too much fat start to take their toll on the heart. Up to that point, men in general have an inadvertently healthier attitude to food. They tend to be more active so will eat more, and, because of the variety of different foods they'll consume, they're more likely to stock up on the kinds of nutrients they need. Women, on the other hand, are more likely to deprive themselves of food in a weight-loss diet and are therefore more likely to miss out on their nutrient quota. In one survey in Australia 35% of women as opposed to 1.3% of men had iron intakes of less than 70% of the recommended level. Iron is particularly important during pregnancy, and again, a good cereal breakfast can not only take care of this, but will provide enough fibre to cure the constipation 38% of pregnant women suffer. 20% of the elderly complain about this problem too, and this could account for the sudden rise in breakfasting in the over-55 age group.

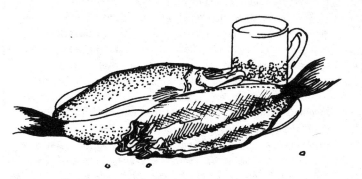

Minerals like iron are the key to looking better, as described in Chapter Two. Healthy hair, teeth, nails and skin are dependent on a good balance of iron, zinc and calcium. Calcium is also vital for combating depression, anxiety, panic attacks, hyperactivity and subsequent insomnia. All these are signs of stress, and sufferers should check that they're getting enough milk, cheese or yoghurt and nuts, dark green leafy vegetables and pulses.

People who eat breakfast are more likely to be getting enough B group vitamins, which were shown in Chapter Two's Swansea study to promote a feeling of well-being. But eating a good breakfast high in fibre and filled with carbohydrates is also likely to lower your fat and cholesterol through the day. An American study examined the breakfast habits and cholesterol levels of over 11,000 adults recently, and found that the daily intake of cholesterol and fats was directly related to their choice of breakfast foods. Cooked breakfasts of eggs, bacon, sausage, ham, pancakes, waffles and French toast – not necessarily all together – massively increased their cholesterol intake. But it also showed that, regardless of the type of food they were eating, people who skipped breakfast completely were found to have an even higher level of cholesterol in the blood.

Worryingly, the American Health Foundation found that this wasn't just the case for adults. In a study of the breakfast habits of 530 schoolchildren, the breakfast skippers also had higher cholesterol levels than their breakfasting friends. And as high cholesterol levels are more often than not found in overweight people, the future looks bleak if America's children don't get their act together. Meanwhile in France, a study of schoolchildren found that those eating larger breakfasts and smaller evening meals maintained a normal weight while obesity was the result of a small breakfast and large evening meal. Even when the calorific content of the foods was exactly the same for both groups, the children who ate more in the first half of the day burnt off more calories. This, the experts decided, was proof positive that a good breakfast can help people to lose weight and to maintain their desired level.

The shot of glucose that breakfast cereals will give you first thing in the morning means you won't be ravenous by lunchtime and will be more capable of making a sensible choice about the food you eat. Again, those regulated blood sugar levels mean that you're not going to be making erratic decisions about chocolate bars in the afternoon and will be more in tune with your body's real needs by the time you choose your evening meal. A low-fat, high-fibre diet is easily kicked off by eating breakfast regularly and, according to all the studies, gives you a head start in basic nutrition. But if you're still in the dark after three chapters of facts about fat and fibre, perhaps you're just one of those unfortunate people whose attention span isn't quite what it should be. In which case, here's the breakfast skipper's guide to becoming a well-rounded individual . . .

THE LOW-FAT HABIT

- Choose low-fat breakfast cereals like Corn Flakes, Special K, Rice Krispies, All-Bran, Bran Flakes, Fruit 'n Fibre, Common Sense, etc.

- Use semi-skimmed, skimmed or fat-free milk.

- Add seasonal fruit to your cereal – berries, kiwi fruit, etc.

- Dried fruit is available all year; figs and dates are particularly high in fibre.

- Use fruit jams and honey instead of butter and margarine on your bread and toast. If you can, buy fresh bread which is moist enough not to have to use a spread.

FOUR

OUT TO LUNCH

In his book *Nature's Gift of Food*, naturopath Jan de Vries tells of how he was visiting a health exhibition with Gloria Hunniford. They came across a stall offering cholesterol testing, and when they tried it, they found that Hunniford's level was lower than his, which came out as above average – a bit embarrassing considering his job is to tell people how to eat healthily. The reason lay in their eating habits; both normally ate a low-fat, high-fibre diet but de Vries had recently been away from home, eating on planes and in hotels where the food tended to be much richer. He immediately boosted his breakfast with oat bran, ate a lot of grapes – including chewing the pips thoroughly – and within a short space of time, his level was back to a more desirable 5.2.

This story will strike at the heart of many business people who feel out of control once they're out of their own kitchen. It's certainly helpful to know your way around your larder in order to be able to plan a healthy daily menu for you and your family but most people most of the time are at the mercy of caterers, whether it's the sandwich shop across the road, British Rail's buffet car or British Airways' galley. If you're away on business more than a couple of times a week, then you could find that your diet is being hijacked.

It's vital when you're away from home on a merry-go-round of business meetings, often in different countries, dealing with a variety of cultures, time zones and foreign food, that you keep your energy levels up to scratch. It may sound glamorous to jet

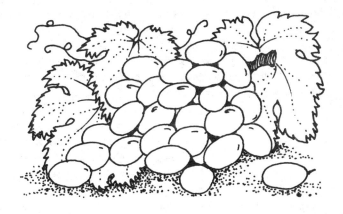

around the world half the year, but the reality can be a nightmare for your heart, your figure and your sleep patterns. It needn't be. Slowly, information is getting through to the caterers on the trains, boats and planes that while we want to be spoilt rotten, we don't have to have Hollandaise sauce with *everything*, vegetarian options don't have to be shuffled out half-heartedly to the odd-looking people in the cheap seats, and just because we're away from home, we *will* still appreciate a healthy breakfast.

Not that the executive chefs at British Rail would believe it if they saw the gang of businessmen on a trip to Leeds on the 07.50 enthusiastically digging in to the Great British Breakfast. 'Well, it's a treat, isn't it?' 32-year-old James, an account executive at an advertising agency told me as he scoffed his bacon, egg, sauté potatoes and black pudding. 'I get enough muesli at home, and want to push the boat out now and again.'

British Rail's executive chef, David Small, explained that they had tried the healthier options. 'We spent a lot of money on yoghurts and muesli and I'm afraid it failed dismally. In two months, we had two takers. The average customer is in a holiday mood when they get on the train, and they want their treats.'

British Rail do offer kippers (drenched in butter, but you can always ask them not to) and smoked salmon and scrambled eggs, as well as cereals, brown rolls and toast. Fresh fruit has already been cut into oxidising little pieces, but is a token effort towards health. Food is oxidised when cells are cut and oxygen is allowed in. Shrink wrapping – or covering in cling film – goes some way to limit the oxygen coming in, but only if it's wrapped tightly around the bowls. If not, fresh fruit which has been cut into a salad will be steadily losing its vitamins, and, if it's sitting around in a train's kitchen for a good few hours, it's not going to be in tip-top condition by the time it gets to your plate. Of course, it's going to do you more good than a grill tray of fried egg and black pudding but you'd be better off following your bread and cereal with a bowl of fresh fruit in its original glory.

If you haven't seen even the oxidised fruit salad on the buffet car list of tariffs, you'll have noticed that British Rail's commitment to token health options doesn't extend to second-class travellers who don't want to pay an arm and a leg in the dining car. Chocolate croissants and egg and cress sandwiches are about as good as it gets in the buffet car. But it's not necessarily British Rail's fault. They have a remit to make a profit and need to rely on the results of surveys to find out what exactly will sell. In a small kitchen, they can't afford to carry food which is not likely to be eaten so the message the customer is giving BR – give us grill trays and bacon and tomato rolls – is the only one to which they will respond.

David Small explains, 'Food and hygiene rules which demand that we keep food in as perfect an environment as possible, as well as profit margins, dictate what we keep on board. We rely completely on knowing our customers' needs better than they do so that we minimise any wastage.' So if you decide not to eat the yoghurts and cereals then they will believe that you don't want them. Of course, if they're not there you have no choice, but caterers will blame the tiny travelling kitchens for the problem. The bacon and tomato roll is their biggest seller in the buffet car and is not a bad way of offering a tasty, nutritious and high-fibre option. The bacon is grilled, the roll is wholemeal and the tomatoes are fresh, all of which will give you a reasonable amount of energy for your trip away.

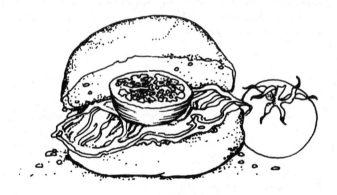

Men seem to act like overgrown schoolboys on a train and believe that because it's just a day trip – or at most a couple of days away from home – they can feast on fats and live to tell the tale. Cholesterol levels are generally watched over by their wives, and, when the boys are out of town, they're likely to eat the breakfasts their mothers made them. The news that the traditional British breakfast is known as 'a heart attack on a plate' – particularly for middle-aged men – hadn't reached their childhood kitchens of the forties, fifties and sixties, and the smell of bacon and eggs can still render a grown man helpless, erasing any scant nutritional knowledge he might have gathered.

On the 07.50 to Leeds, most men were eating the full grill-tray breakfast, including black pudding, while the handful of women in the First Class and Dining Car were tucking into cereals and toast or fish. Barbara, a civil servant in her thirties, was eating scrambled eggs and salmon. She told me she didn't like fried food, had been up since 5 a.m. and couldn't face much at that time of the morning. Her colleague, Paul, was thrilled with his grill tray. 'I love to treat myself at other people's expense,' he grinned. 'I don't feel bad about this at all because normally I'd have muesli when I'm at home and I reckon that makes me pretty good.'

The Grill Tray	Fat	Fibre	Calories
grilled back bacon (25g)	4.7	–	73
pork sausage (35g)	8.6	–	111.3
scrambled egg (120g)	27	–	296
mushrooms (boiled) (44g)	0.1	0.6	4.8
black pudding (30g)	6.57	–	91.5
sauté potatoes (100g)	4.5	1.8	149
fried bread (30g)	9.6	0.5	151
	61.2g	2.9g	877 kc

This idea of 'good' versus 'naughty' foods seemed to be the predominant factor in most people's choice. David Small confirms that, from his surveys, this is the way that most Britons see food. But the 'schoolboys' seem to grow up when they travel by plane. Airlines are much more in touch with our needs when we're crossing time zones, our feet are swelling and the last thing our stomachs need is a rich sauce and fatty meat. American Airlines have begun to consult customers about their health requirements, and to talk to some of the country's most popular chefs about changing trends. The answer seems to be in preparing a smaller choice of better food which is tailor-made to suit the needs of the long-haul traveller. And they're not alone. Most airlines are now taking measures not only to keep up with their more demanding and sophisticated traveller but also to keep one step ahead of their increasingly nutrition-conscious competition. British Airways have taken the un-precedented step of looking to the East for some revolutionary ideas about food, the body and relaxation. Club World and First Class travellers are able to try this out on long-haul trips, and Economy passengers should write to BA and encourage them to extend it to the back of the plane.

The idea is to get you to your destination fit and alert, and bring you home rested and refreshed. 'Well Being in the Air' is the brainchild of BA's Kurt Haffner. 'There's so much we didn't know about what happens to your body at altitude,' he told me, 'and we used to just put up with the effects of jet lag, swelling and dehydration. But our medical staff, including physio-therapists and nutritionists who have been looking after our cabin crews for years, have accumulated a huge amount of knowledge about what eating and exercise can do for your state of mind, and know now what to offer our customers.'

Jim Dunlop, BA's head of health services, explains what happens at altitude. 'Flying at thirty thousand feet means it's actually sub-zero low-pressure hell out there, and, although the cabin pressure is much higher, it's still equivalent to being at about six to eight thousand feet.' That's like being at the top of the average mountain, and means your body is getting 25 per cent less oxygen than it's used to. It's not harmful – there are plenty of people who live on mountains higher than

8,000 feet – but there's going to be much less air pressure weighing down on you than if you were at sea level, and your body expands automatically. Hence the swelling we experience in the air, as well as the blocked sinuses and pressure in the ears. Loose clothing is the answer, as well as taking shoes off during the flight. If you're on business and your firm is paying a First Class fare you'll even get a sleeper suit and duvet after 7 p.m.

Jim Dunlop points out that alcohol and caffeine are likely to give you a headache at altitude and make you sluggish. 'Lots of plain water or fruit juice is the best bet.' Fizzy water at altitude will become even more gassy in your stomach and will lead to more swelling. The right food is vital. Carbohydrates are the easiest food group to digest, using less energy for processing in the body and so making it easier to relax and sleep after the meal. The Well Being programme has therefore based its menu on lots of pasta, rice and potato dishes with minimum dairy products and meat. Fibre is essential if you're going to keep your system regular while you're away and is one of the ideal food groups to eat at altitude.

Low salt is one of the keys to fighting dehydration in the dry cabin air. Dehydration can be one of the main contributors to jet lag. The best way to beat it is to make sure you don't drink too much alcohol during the flight, and then to take some aerobic exercise when you land. Rotating your head in your seat, flexing and relaxing muscles and walking around the cabin will also help you sleep when you finally get to bed, but swimming or a long walk when you reach your destination is unbeatable. Jim Dunlop explains, 'It speeds up your body's metabolism so it can settle down faster whatever time zone you've crossed into.'

Jet lag is caused by your mind and body failing to adapt to new rhythms of light and sleep. Dr Aric Sigman was a consultant on the Well Being programme and explains that the best

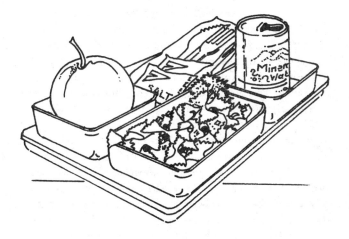

psychological way to beat jet lag is to think yourself into the time zone you're going to. 'Set your watch to the new time while you're still in the air and when you get there, eat your meals when everyone else is eating theirs. Get lots of exposure to natural light, sleep in the local time pattern, and you'll find that business trips will cease to be a nightmare.'

I tried it out. I had to go to New York for three days, had four interviews to do – all on different subjects – so had to keep my head together. I'd be having lunch with business colleagues every day and dinner with friends every night. My schedule when I got back home was also going to be tight, so I couldn't afford to be bed bound. A schedule like this is hardly unusual, but if your body is having to deal with a different time zone and eating patterns, as well as the stress of the business meetings themselves, it needs to be treated with even more reverence than usual.

On the flight out I asked a number of Business and First Class travellers for their tips for a successful trip. The few macho travellers who fly very regularly (and looked particularly haggard) said that they didn't really pay much attention to what they ate and drank, while many of the women weren't eating at all. They told me that they were so concerned about their diet that they ate before they got on board. A bit excessive perhaps, but, from experience of doing a five-day business trip to New York every month, one woman said that it was the only way.

It's no use being well prepared for your arrival if you then spend the week pigging out on fatty foods. Food can be one of the real perks of a business trip, and most countries offer plenty of great local dishes which won't weigh you down. From Singapore to Sydney, you'll be able to take advantage of the many different ethnic influences whose cuisine follows the low-fat, high-fibre ideal. Eating sushi for a couple of days in Tokyo will send you home positively brimming with health. New York is probably better suited to the healthy eater than most cities in America with its cornucopia of delicatessens and restaurants. The Italian community didn't wait for the Mediterranean diet to become fashionable before offering its customers a mouth-watering selection of olive oils, pasta and imaginative fish dishes. Remember that it's chiefly only in Northern Europe and America that people have been keeling over from diet-related diseases for the past 50 years, and that much of the local cooking from the Mediterranean through Africa to South America and the Far East has stuck to its original recipe for health for thousands of years.

Even the big hotels which used to be notorious for pandering to the culinary whim of the over-indulgent Western business person are beginning to change their attitude. Most hotels in cities with an international business market can't afford to lag behind the nutritional initiative many chains are now taking. The international Hyatt chain, for example, is promoting a range they call cuisine naturelle which will soon be in operation throughout the world. Incorporated into the Hyatt's standard menu, it offers low-fat, high-fibre foods which are designed specifically for business lunches. Their chefs understand that the rise in glucose levels after a big meal, as the body works overtime to digest it all, means that concentration levels fall and however important that business meeting is, all the body wants is a snooze. Cuisine naturelle is careful to use only a teaspoon of oil and organically grown fruit and vegetables as well as special fat-free cuts of meat and fresh herbs.

This initiative came from the results of a report by the American National Restaurant Association which said that 55% of diners rate nutrition as their top concern but still choose food for its taste; 40% of business travellers said that they felt eating healthily was a priority when they were away from home. Robert Dallain, the vice president of catering for the Hyatt chain, sums up this new attitude: 'More and more meetings are held with health, relaxation and recreation in mind, but the emphasis has always been on the activities rather than the food. We're seeing meetings with lots of spa treatments and exercise time, but with high-fat, high-cholesterol meals to top it all off. It's a self-defeating process.' What the Hyatt has done is to take popular though not necessarily healthy dishes like French toast, and prepare them with a minimum of fat and maximum of taste (see page 167 for recipes). Nutritionist Pam Smith was the consultant to the programme and suggests a high-fibre breakfast such as whole-wheat pancakes to jump-start the body and make sure you don't get hunger pangs in the middle of your morning meeting. She also goes along with the nibbling theory outlined in Chapter Two. 'A mid-morning snack to "re-energise" the body should be something like fresh fruits, low-fat cheeses, low-fat muffins, breads and yoghurts instead of the standard high-fat Danishes and croissants.'

Perhaps for the business person who ordinarily wouldn't get home until past 9 p.m., a business dinner is no bad thing. They tend to be at more reasonable hours of the evening so the hosts can get home. As the body's metabolism slows down towards the end of the day, it becomes harder to work off a big meal after the early evening, and some experts recommend that we don't eat after 6 p.m. One of the most successful weight-loss tips for people who like their food and will not cut down on portions is not to eat a morsel after 7 p.m., and to go for a walk after dinner. Cutting down on fat and increasing fibre will obviously make a bigger difference, but simply by tuning into the body's metabolic rate the food has time to be digested properly and burnt off before bed.

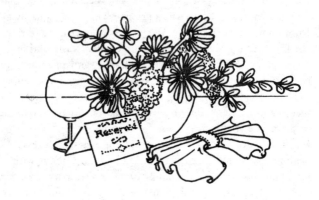

A quick trip around the most popular business hotels showed the changing trend; the Millenium, which has recently opened opposite the World Trade Center in New York, offers an almost exclusively Mediterranean menu. 'Food used to be very old fashioned Downtown,' Kathleen Duffy of the Millenium told me. 'We used to eat lots of fish, because we're so near the bay, but also steaks by the ton. Men used to be in the majority in the financial sector here but when women started to join them for the business lunches, they had the most profound influence.' Women weren't just eager to keep their stomachs flat while wheeling and dealing; they wanted to keep their heads clear while their male colleagues relied on getting their clients to loosen up over a bottle of wine. These same women were almost certainly unaware that the vegetables and salads they were munching into had as much to do with the clarity of their argument as the sparkling mineral water did.

Eating a diet that's low in fat and high in fibre is essential while you're away, and especially if you've crossed the time zone. Fat actually inhibits the secretion of gastric juices which upsets the body's chemistry, making it difficult to digest properly and leaving you constipated. Fibre makes sure you stay regular; the last thing you need is to feel sluggish, a frequent symptom of constipation. Breakfast for most people is possibly the only meal of the day when they're thinking about their inner health. Many find that they have to have the same breakfast every day if they're to stay regular, and despite the cereals and breads available in my hotels, I wish I'd taken my Fruit 'n Fibre.

BRITAIN BITES BACK

A growing band of chefs has changed the shape of the British menu and is encouraging foreign visitors to think again about dismissing British cooking as no more interesting than fish and chips. And it's not just the gurus of haute cuisine who are presenting the wholegrain rolls with sun dried tomatoes, the pastas and polentas with Sicilian sauces and the roasted vegetable salads drizzled with extra virgin olive oil. Many chefs who do not charge a fortune for their imaginative and extremely healthy dishes have revolutionised the business of eating out – with or without your clients.

Le Meridien Hotel in Piccadilly boasts that its Oak Room is one of the best dining-rooms in London, but, in these recessionary days, recognises that business lunches have to be more economical, and serves great food at more realistic prices in the Garden Terrace. Head chef David Chambers knows that his customers are also more likely to be concerned about their health than they used to be and appreciates the challenge set him by Le Meridien's nutrition guru, Jacques Manière. Like many great chefs, Manière believes in the words of nineteenth-century French philosopher Brillat-Savarin when he wrote 'you are what you eat', and he developed the great man's ideas about the power of steam to bring out the best in food.

In his book *Le Grand Livre de la Cuisine à la Vapeur* (*The Encyclopedia of Steam Cookery*) Manière explained how nutritionists had worked against the advance of good cooking: around 1930, a new science had developed and was being imposed on the public. But 'La Diététique' – the strict eating regime which doctors would recommend to patients with heart problems – split the world of food in two, with chefs and lovers of cooking on one side and scientists on the other. If you've ever seen one of those doctors' diets, you'll know what the chefs were worried about: food was to be stripped down to its very basics with very few suggestions about how to make boiled potatoes and chicken interesting or tasty. While fat was out and 'roughage' (as fibre used to be called) was in, nobody told us what to do with what was left in our food cupboards. Food was the enemy once again, and while restaurants refused to play ball with the nutritionists, haute cuisine became a temptress for the millions of patients who had to make do with rabbit food. Once they'd done their six-week diet the patients were almost bound to fall back into the pattern of indulgence and denial which had probably caused their problem in the first place.

The chefs argued on, Manière leading the way and insisting that there had to be a meeting of minds if people who liked food could expect to live beyond middle age. Vegetables which could play a key role in healthy cuisine were supposed to be cooked rapidly so that vitamins and minerals would be left intact, said the nutritionists, but chefs wanted space to be able to roast, steam or sauté them if the recipe required it. Fat added taste, the chefs argued – but increased cholesterol, the scientists pointed out.

Desperate attempts were made to meet in the middle, until finally 'nouvelle cuisine' was developed, using many of the principles both camps were happy with. But the public weren't. For a while, back in the eighties, we put up with nasturtiums on a vast white plate but it wasn't long before the hungry came out of the closet and asked for their food back. Jacques Manière was one of the chefs to lead the revolt. He pointed to a type of cooking the Chinese had been doing since the beginning of time but which was largely undiscovered in Europe until the Algerian immigrants of the fifties and sixties brought their methods of making couscous to France. Steam was introduced to haute cuisine and pioneered a whole new way of cooking for the health-conscious foodie.

Manière's cuisine à la vapeur means steam-cooking fish, meat or vegetables on a bed of herbs and onions or shallots and garlic. No fat is used, but more importantly for the foodie, the delicacy of taste is kept intact. At Le Meridien's Garden Terrace restaurant, I sliced into my lamb cutlet, amazed that steam could produce such a delicate piece of meat. Perfectly pink, it melted in my mouth and laid barely an ounce of cholesterol on my arteries. The fat on the meat was cut off in the preparation, and the process of steaming encourages any extra fat to fall out of the meat. Of course, some fat will stay in any meat in order for it to remain succulent, but by reducing it so dramatically and still producing such a tasty dish you're getting the best of both worlds.

David Chambers, whose Michelin star for Le Meridien's Oak Room shows how well he has incorporated the principles of his mentor Manière into his cooking, feels that it would be more difficult to promote high-fibre dishes. 'The whole thing about haute cuisine is finesse,' he explains. 'With the trend towards low fat, you can prepare light delicate dishes like the steamed lamb, but fibre by its very nature is coarse. Having said that, we serve great wholemeal rolls, and a low-fat dish will always lend itself to having lots of barely cooked vegetables. They won't be served in their skins, so the fibre will be reduced, but in terms of giving the customer a few ideas about how to cook delicious healthy dishes, I think we're on the right track.'

However, lentilles de puy – the green lentils which are packed with fibre – do lend themselves to fine dining. Chambers prepared a dish of lentilles de puy cooked for 20 minutes in duck stock with steamed celeriac, onions, carrots and leeks which was delicious. He explains that lentils can be cooked in the stock of whatever you're serving them with – fish, chicken, beef – but stresses that it's only the green lentils which are delicate enough for these kinds of dishes. 'I've served them with duck with truffle sauce,' said Chambers. 'I've even stuffed a cabbage and filo pastry with them. Anything is possible with a green lentil.'

One of the interesting changes in good restaurants in recent years has been the growth in selection of bread rolls. Once upon a time not too long ago, bread was something on which we filled up while we waited for our starter. But with raisin bread, poppy-seed-encrusted rolls and walnuts poking out of your wholegrain bap, you're on your way to a fabulous feast of fibre before you've even got to the lentils. Take London's Soho Soho, a restaurant which has successfully merged the concept of health and great cooking. Owner Lawrence Isaacson suffered from worryingly high cholesterol in his blood a couple of years ago, but, an avid foodie and regular business luncher, he couldn't bear the thought of dining out on boiled potatoes and tasteless grilled chicken. When his doctor advised him to follow a more Mediterranean-style diet, using olive oil, red wine and fibre to reduce his cholesterol level, he decided to open a restaurant for all those people like him who wanted to eat out, but eat well. The menus explain exactly what's in a dish so that customers can not only make sure that they're eating the right oil and enough fibre, but be inspired enough to try the dishes at home. But it's the rolls which are one of Soho Soho's most inspiring ideas and they don't even appear on the menu. Next time you're baking bread, throw in a couple of olives, or sun dried tomatoes, and sprinkle them with poppy seeds. Your fibre levels will shoot up and you'll never be satisfied with white sliced again . . .

Even for the non-foodie who likes to go for a bite with friends, eating out need not be a nutritional lucky dip. In fact, one cancer study suggests that the more you eat with friends, the less likely you may be to get cancer. This study, which is still running in the States, is looking at the possible promoters of cancer from our lifestyle, and has discovered that the lowest incidence of the disease is found among people who are more sociable. While the study is still inconclusive, scientist John Cairns believes that by eating a wider variety of foods in a less stressful environment the possible dangers from certain foods are diluted. 'If you have more friends,' he explained, 'you're more likely to eat Indian one night, Chinese another, or more homecooked food at people's houses. If there was a potentially carcinogenic substance in any particular food, you're not going to be subjecting yourself to too much of it because you're eating so many different things.' He also thought it could have something to do with a more relaxed environment for your digestion which allows the body's defence system to get what it needs from the nutrients in food. He was keen to point out that this doesn't amount to conclusive evidence. 'There's no harm in being more sociable in the fight against cancer though,' he said. 'At least you'll have more fun . . .'

Study after study suggests that low self-esteem, stress and deprivation can provide a breeding ground for cancers. For the person who has been imprisoned by diets for most of their adult life this advice has never been so welcome. The message from experts is to get wise about the food you eat, and then use it to choose the best food at the supermarket, in your favourite restaurants and in the kitchen.

THE EATING OUT GUIDE

- Look at the menu before you go in. If it's full of creamy sauces, you can bet the chef hasn't got a great imagination. Pastas with tomato sauces are much tastier.

- Grilled meat and fish doesn't have to be the dieter's option alone. If it's smothered in herbs and marinated in olive oil, it's going to be extremely good for you and very tasty too.

- Vegetable dishes are some of the most interesting at the moment. If a chef doesn't know what to do with them, it might be worth saving your money.

- Lentils and pulses taste wonderful across Africa, India and the Mediterranean, but only the most imaginative British chefs have caught on. Why not show some of the recipes in this book to your local chefs and boost fibre levels across town?

Waiters are also taking advantage of the culinary revolution and playing a much more active role in advising their customers about the food. Don't be afraid to ask them whether something has been cooked in oil or butter, and whether you can have your fish or chicken grilled rather than fried. They'll appreciate the fact that you're involving them rather than using them as your servant for the evening. You'll find that you'll get a better response from both waiter and chef if you take an interest in the food they're preparing. And if you find that they can't be bothered with your questions, get stroppy; it is your money after all . . .

Of course there are times when you want to indulge and until we realise that healthy food doesn't have to taste of cardboard, we'll associate eating out with pigging out. Eugene McCoy, of McCoys Tontine in Staddlebridge, Cleveland, says that his Mediterranean favourites are the least popular on his bistro menu. 'My brother Tom can cook what he likes in the restaurant upstairs,' he said, 'but what I cook for the bistro customer is down to what sells. This area is very tough and the people are stubborn in their ways, so we have to rely on cooking simple dishes with the best possible ingredients and stick on a couple of frilly corners. Take the Mediterranean prawns which we marinate with garlic, capsicum and capers; we'll sell two tonight, and the rest will go for the steak au poivre. People like creamy sauces around here – they go for what they wouldn't necessarily cook at home.' However, despite having to go heavy on the cream on occasion, Eugene's menu reads like something straight out of Provence. His cooking is not inspired by health advice, but by the great tastes of the South of France; yet because he uses extra virgin olive oil, and in spite of the fact that his pulses and lentils may not be specifically designed to boost Cleveland's fibre intake, he's doing wonders for the energy levels in Staddlebridge . . .

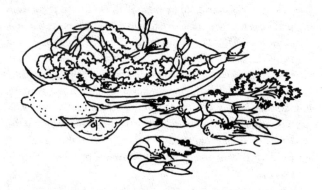

Eating great food needn't cost a fortune either. Britain has become much more cosmopolitan over the last decade, with Greek, Lebanese, Italian, Indian, Thai, Spanish and Turkish restaurants springing up in just about every town. The bigger cities are now bursting with a plethora of vegetarian restaurants where you'll find some of the more interesting and imaginative dishes at the bottom end of the price range. Britain may have only just discovered that food is the key to good health of body and mind, but the chefs who present us with hummus, fish kebabs marinated in olive oil, garlic and rosemary, artichokes and fresh broad beans with lemon juice and grilled marinated vegetable salad come from countries where it's been taken for granted since the beginning of time.

Puddings are a different matter. Maddalena Bonino, chef at Covent Garden's Bertorelli's, grew up in rural Italy feeding her diabetic father the best 'healing' food the countryside had to offer. But puddings, she says, have more benefit on the spirit. 'Normally Italians don't eat them,' she told me. 'After a meal, we drink coffee and maybe eat some fruit, and on special occasions we eat the most wonderful cakes. We see it as pure indulgence and appreciate it so much more if we keep it to special days like Sundays, or birthdays. So there's no such thing as a healthy pudding – they must be full of cream – what's the point otherwise?'

Luckily, while most of us agree, there are plenty of healthier options on the menus of most restaurants these days. Business lunches are probably responsible for the change; a combination of the influence of more figure-conscious women, and over-stressed men who have been warned by their doctors, has once again thrown out the challenge to chefs. Fruit is the healthiest way of finishing a meal, and now that we can get just about

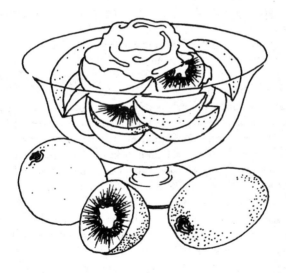

anything all year round in the supermarket we're spoilt for choice in many restaurants. Cream has been pushed aside to make way for lower fat fromage frais and yoghurts. Fruit can be baked, grilled, flambéd, and souffléd, served with sorbets, red, white and dessert wines, with olive oil biscuits, stuffed with other fruits, low-fat cream cheeses or nuts, and rolled in oats, yoghurt and honey to make the most filling of desserts, and all of them low in fat and high in fibre.

Even stopping off at the sandwich shop needn't be a reason to stray from your new regime. In fact sandwiches of wholemeal bread with a variety of fresh salads, tuna or other fish, grilled meats and fresh vegetables like tomatoes, spinach or cucumber are extremely good ways of boosting your fibre intake while getting a delicious, cheap and easy lunch. Obviously, drowning the whole lot in high-fat mayonnaise won't do much for the waistline, and you can always ask for a polyunsaturated margarine, or a low-fat spread or, even better, use olive oil – instead of butter. The choice is completely yours in a sandwich shop – provided it has a reasonable selection of fillings, and you can oversee the whole procedure.

Fresh bread is moist enough not to need any butter or margarine, and if it's packed with extra nuts and grains it'll not only taste better but send your fibre levels rocketing. Baked potatoes are also extremely good sources of fibre, with most of it in the skin. You can get them from most sandwich bars for a very reasonable price. Have them filled with tuna, sweetcorn or baked beans for a low-fat, high-fibre lunch. Some people think that they are too dry without lashings of butter or mayonnaise, but try olive oil and you'll be hooked for life.

The fast food giants seem to have lured a whole generation away from real food despite having the money and the means to encourage an interest in nutrition. A beefburger with salad and chips is in itself not a bad meal. If only the bun were bigger and brown with more fibre, the salad contained more than a bit of gherkin and half a tomato, the chips were wider and hadn't absorbed so much fat, and the whole lot wasn't drowned in mayonnaise. Making your own beefburgers take no time at all; you could get your kids to help, encouraging them from an early age that fast food isn't about ordering, buying and eating it as quickly as possible, but about great smells emanating from

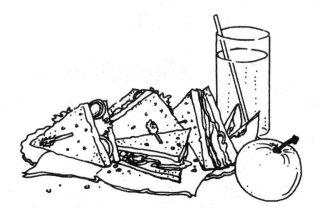

the kitchen and delicious, crunchy burgers that are good for you.

But at least fast food is the final frontier in the battle to restore our reputation for good food in this country. Have a look at the recipes in the back of this book and arm yourself with facts to throw at the next tourist who complains about British food. We may have fallen behind the rest of the world in the last fifty years, but we're now in a prime position to copy the best of what it has to offer.

FIVE

THE WESTERN DISEASES

The fact that our society has spawned the people who were responsible for penicillin, the telephone and Cat's-eyes makes us look even more stupid for killing ourselves by eating badly. We could forgive the rest of the world for thinking that, as a nation, we might have a deathwish, with heart disease at epidemic proportions and the biggest cause of premature death in this country, and cancer – particularly of the bowel and breast – following close behind. One in five people in Britain die from diet-related diseases. It would be embarrassing if it weren't so tragic, as well as being such a drain on the economy; the National Health Service spends £500 million a year on entirely preventable illnesses and, in 1992, the Department of Health called a halt to this outrageous trend, recommending strict nutritional guidelines. In this, the most disturbing of chapters, we take a closer look at some of those diseases which can, given the right diet, be helped to be prevented at the earliest stage.

CANCER

Cancer is the second biggest killer after coronary heart disease, and, sadly, one in three people can expect to develop it in some form.

Since Dr Denis Burkitt's breakthrough studies in Africa in the seventies, when he discovered the correlation between cancer and lack of fibre in the diet, a vast amount of research has been done. The Imperial Cancer Research Fund alone needs £40 million per annum to spend on research to reverse the cancer trend. Epidemiologists Sir Richard Doll and Richard Peto produced a ground-breaking document in 1981 which concluded that 80% of cancers were potentially avoidable and that diet played a significant role in 35% of them. High fat, alcohol and animal protein consumption, they found, were possible promoters of cancer but, perhaps more importantly, they discovered that a wide variety of foods would inhibit it.

They've concluded that food is definitely one of the keys to unlocking a whole host of cancer-prevention methods, but in the meantime we spend a fortune on shutting the door after the horse has bolted. 'An early diagnosis is never going to reduce the numbers,' explained Dr Burkitt. 'The answer is quite simple – too much money is going into the treatment rather than the prevention of cancer.'

We still don't understand enough about cancer. So far we know categorically that smoking causes cancer, that we shouldn't have too many sexual partners without using protection, that obesity can be a causal factor, and that we shouldn't get sunburnt. We know that fruit, vegetables and cereals have a beneficial effect but we are still very unclear about other important dietary factors. Early evidence is emerging from America to suggest that fats might not be as big a problem in promoting cancers as *fatness*. Heart disease *is* caused by too much saturated fat, however, so this evidence, even it were found to be the case, shouldn't change our low-fat habit. Epidemiologists, the scientists who carefully monitor human behaviour over long periods of time in order to study the contexts within which, for example, we eat, drink or have sex, are careful to wait until the end of their studies before making wild claims. If it looks like high-fat diets are *not* the main problem behind breast cancer, then the other common elements of the test group – of nurses in this particular American study – must be scrutinised. Obesity seems to be the main contributor to many cancers, and nurses have also been shown to drink a lot of alcohol. While alcohol itself might not be the cause, drinking too much and putting on too much weight could well be.

In 1991, the world's largest ever in-depth study of the relationship between diet and cancer was launched, with seven European countries looking at the eating and living habits of 250,000 people over ten years. France, Germany, Greece, Italy, the Netherlands and Spain are taking part in this study (known as EPIC), which will cost £2 million in Britain alone. In Britain, 85,000 people are allowing their lifestyles to be scrutinised and their blood and urine samples to be regularly tested, and scientists predict that, of that test group, 4,000 will develop some form of cancer in the next ten years. The epidemiologists should be able to make enough comparisons between those affected by cancer in all seven countries right across Europe to be able to pin down the common causes of a number of different cancers.

Breast and bowel cancer will be the first to be investigated, being two of the major killers in the Western world. Stomach, prostate, pancreas, cervical, ovarian and bladder cancers will then be put under the microscope as information about the first two emerges. The roles of fat and fibre as potential contributor and preventor will be the first dietary components to be looked at. Scotland has already come up with a recommendation of how its own cancer statistics can be changed by eating differently:

CANCER DEATHS POSSIBLY AVOIDABLE BY DIETARY CHANGE IN SCOTLAND

Cancer	Total number	% Avoidable
large bowel	1,737	90%
breast	1,250	50%
stomach	877	90%
prostate	645	10%
pancreas	642	50%
all cancers	14,957	35%

(Source: Scottish Health Statistics 1991. Scottish Health Service, Edinburgh)

In the meantime, the Imperial Cancer Research Fund which is participating in the EPIC study has issued this clear dietary guide to reducing the risk of stomach cancer. Bearing in mind how careful they are to cross-reference every study over many years, this information can be seen as reliable.

- Increased fresh fruit and vegetable intake decreases the risk of stomach cancer
- People with moderate levels of intake, for example one piece of fruit a day, have 30–50% less risk
- If the entire population had a similar intake 17–33% of stomach cancers could be prevented

COLORECTAL CANCER

Colorectal cancer accounts for 12% of all cancer deaths in Britain. It is unique in that polyps, or wart-like growths in the colon, are found up to 15 years before cancer develops. It tends to affect the middle-aged and elderly, and is quite difficult to catch in its early stages because the symptoms are vague and might include nothing more than abnormal bowel habits or slight abdominal discomfort.

Red meat and animal fat as well as a low intake of fibre are associated with the development of the polyp while wheatbran seems to stop it developing into cancer. The bile acids at work in the colon are made into secondary bile acids as they are reabsorbed into the bloodstream. But these secondary acids may be carcinogens which, if left too long in the colon through constipation, will start to interfere with cell reproduction – the very first stage in the development of cancer. By eating more fibre, nature's broom simply sweeps them into the faecal pile of waste and sends them out of the body in a nice big stool. The regular action of sweeping the system clean makes the colon a thoroughly undesirable environment for carcinogens to do their worst.

Dr Jerome de Cosse of the Memorial-Sloan Kettering Cancer Centre found that these precancerous growths in the colon could actually be shrunk by two ordinary (30g each) servings of All-Bran a day. It also acted to slow the progress of the development of the polyp into the cancerous tumour, all of which suggests that it's not necessarily too late – even if you've already got a growth – to do something about it.

It's not just our bodies which have to be in excellent condition to fight disease, but also the food we feed them. It needs to be as unbruised and undissected as possible by the time it reaches our lips so that oxygen can't get into its cells and eat up all its goodness. This process is called oxidation: when food cells are cut an apple or potato, for example, will discolour, showing the effect of the oxygen getting in. If it discolours, it's letting you know that it's not all it might be nutritionally. Our bodies have their own army of anti-oxidants which we make ourselves to fight the free radical activity which attacks the cells in both the food and the body. They are our most important ally in the fight against cancers.

If we eat too much oxidised food without enough natural anti-oxidants – and think about how many foods we cut up before cooking them – the body immediately goes up a gear to compensate. If we eat healthily, we'll maintain a plentiful supply of anti-oxidants, but if the body's own anti-oxidants are used up and not replenished by those in foods like fruit and vegetables, the gloves are off and it's anyone's battle. The free radicals which enter the body with the oxygen are likely to cause havoc with cells and we now know that this can be the launch pad for cancer.

There are a host of anti-oxidants in food, from selenium, found in anything grown in the ground, to olive oil and herbs. Phytate, which is found in high fibre foods, is thought to be an anti-carcinogen, and is extremely effective in squashing these free radicals. Scientists at the University of Maryland have blocked cancer in animals by giving them phytate, and there are several studies which show that it is this rather than the soluble fibre in legumes like beans that reduces cholesterol. To you and me, it doesn't make much difference *what* part of a bean stops cancer and heart disease – let's just *eat* them.

CONSTIPATION

Dr Burkitt discovered that Africans, who were eating two or three times the amount of fibre we consume, were excreting it between 12 and 36 hours later. Compare that with the two to three days our food spends in our system on average – with some elderly people having to put up with it staying around for as long as two weeks. A high-fibre diet relieves constipation almost instantly. Insoluble fibre such as that found in whole-grain cereals is better than the soluble fibre in pulses and vegetables in that it absorbs water like a sponge, and makes the faeces much larger and softer, allowing them to pass out of the system more easily. The straining that has resulted in millions of people suffering from haemorrhoids would become a thing of the past if they ate a little more wholegrain cereal for breakfast.

Some people have a bowel movement no more than three times a week but would not call themselves constipated. How-ever, being regular is more than just a health need; one of life's greatest pleasures must surely be starting every day with a bowel movement. We know that $3\frac{1}{2}$–4 million people in Britain don't have that peace of mind and many more suffer in silence. Constipation affects 20% of the elderly population, 38% of pregnant women and can lead to many of the diseases listed in this chapter.

Bowel movements are not exactly well observed in this country, so very little information exists about what's normal or not. Curiously one of the few studies to have been carried out concentrated on the toilet habits of postmen, nurses, students, old people and men in prison. In the States, one study involved researchers doing a door-to-door survey. The res-ponse to their doorstep question of 'How often do you usually have a bowel movement?' was met with understandable reti-cence, encouraged a lot of white lies, and was dismissed as having little scientific relevance.

Dr Ken Heaton at the University of Bristol decided to fill the void and to try to get a picture of the average British stool: 838 men and 1,059 women from the population of East Bristol were asked to keep strict records of how many times they went to the loo during the week, as well as the shape and size of their stools. And if you'd like to join in at home, the questionnaire asked them to tick one of the following stool types:

1 – Separate hard lumps, like nuts
2 – Sausage-shaped but lumpy
3 – Like a sausage or snake but with cracks on its surface
4 – Like a sausage or snake, smooth and soft
5 – Soft blobs with clear cut edges
6 – Fluffy pieces with ragged edges, a mushy stool

The frequency of defecation wasn't as much of a give-away about internal health as the type of stool. Number one's separate hard lumps were the least desirable, and number six the best sign of a clean colon. Numbers 1–5 mean that you should be eating more insoluble fibre which pushes the food through more quickly, and number six means you've got your diet right. The mushier and bigger the stool, the quicker the transit time of the food passing through the body. The quicker the transit time, the less likelihood of free-radical damage in the intestine – in other words, if the food moves swiftly through the body, there's no time for the baddies to, literally, stick around.

It emerged that men were generally more regular than women, with many of them defecating once a day, inspecting the results more and finding them to be sausage or snake-like in form. Women were more likely to have an irregular bowel movement, sometimes less than five times a week, and passed lumpier, smaller stools. Many people had difficulty in assessing the shape of their stools which is hardly surprising since the design of most British toilet bowls, unlike German ones, for example, encourages stools to sink out of sight. The overwhelming majority of both men and women defecated between seven and nine in the morning. Older women had more problems than women under 50, and it was concluded that they had a slower intestinal transit time.

The most consistent finding in the Bristol study was that women's bowel function is different from men's. Perhaps this is due to the fact that more men are in paid employment and have a more regular schedule than women who may have different pressures such as children to deal with, giving them precious little time to go to the loo when they actually need to. Lower self-esteem has been linked to irregular bowel movements, something else that women tend to suffer from more than men. There could be some hormonal link, although Dr Heaton could not draw any firm conclusions on that one.

The other surprise was that there seems to be no evidence to suggest that we're more likely to get more constipated as we get older. However, the oldest test group was only 60–69: the more active people of this age are, the less likely they are to have a bad diet and exercise pattern. This in turn means that they are more likely to have a regular bowel movement. But there was no notable difference at all in the transit time of the older group from the younger men and women in the Bristol study, and this was a revelation to Dr Heaton and his team of experts.

The most striking finding was that the majority of Britons are not regular. While they may not go so far as to call themselves constipated, there are a lot of people who are feeling more than a little uncomfortable, and the overwhelming majority of them are women of childbearing age. Constipation is not a disease but a symptom of something which has gone wrong – a poor diet, stress, even not drinking enough water. People can suffer from it because they might be in too much of a rush to make time to go to the loo, or, as in the case of many elderly people, they can't be bothered. Being away on business and disrupting your regular schedule, staying in someone else's house, or feeling embarrassed at lack of privacy can all be traumatic enough to bring on constipation.

A good high-fibre breakfast, lots of water throughout the day and plenty of fruit and vegetables will solve most of these problems. A fast, large bowel movement means an end to thumbing through magazines and emerging from your host's loo with a red face and distended stomach.

GALLSTONES

The gall-bladder is a pear-shaped sac attached to the liver which stores and concentrates bile to digest the fat we eat. Fatty foods stimulate the production of a hormone which forces the gall-bladder to contract, forcing the bile into the intestine where fat is absorbed. Too much fatty food can overdo this process and the bile will crystallise and form gallstones.

Most people tend to associate gallstones with obesity, and it is true that if you are overweight you are more likely to secrete more cholesterol into the bile which makes it harder to empty the gall-bladder. Men generally are less prone to them. Most sufferers are female, fair, fat and forty, but Dr Ken Heaton at the University of Bristol has come up with evidence to show that they're not uncommon in the slimmer woman. His study focused in particular on women who were of a normal weight, and found that it came down to a slower intestinal transit time – in other words their food was staying too long in the body before passing out. Women with gallstones and women without, both of normal weight for their height, had their toilet habits closely monitored and their whole-gut transit time measured to see how long it took for them to get rid of their food. The gallstone sufferers' stool output was also significantly lower and their transit time was much slower.

There are several interesting stories about how to get rid of your gallstones, but it's a good idea to check with your doctor first. A diet of fibre and lemon juice has been said to break them down into iridescent green crystals which can be passed with the help of a laxative. The creator of the *Guardian*'s Biff cartoon, Mick Kidd, was 42 and eating a lot of saturated fat in butter, cream and fatty meat when he found that he was suffering from gallstones. Mick wanted to see if there were any alternatives to an operation to remove them, and when an acupuncturist showed him an article about 'the olive oil flush' which was supposed to flush the whole lot out, he wanted to know more. A herbal practitioner confirmed that this was possible by drinking a bottle of olive oil – bit by bit – until the stones pass through. Sure enough, Mick found that the stones did pass, and even had an X-ray to satisfy the doctors that it had worked.

IRRITABLE BOWEL SYNDROME

IBS is often referred to as 'colonic irritation' or 'spastic colon' and is characterised by the unpredictable and urgent need to go to the loo, or by long frustrating bouts of constipation. It's another of the problems from which an extraordinary number of people in the West suffer, and can be relieved by a diet high in fibre. It need involve no other sign of infection or physical cause such as bowel cancer, and no structural damage to the bowel itself. Some sufferers have diarrhoea all the time while others are almost permanently constipated. Most have a stomach ache which is relieved when they have a bowel movement, but others don't. Flatulence, too, is no laughing matter for thousands of people and is often relieved rather than caused by extra fibre in the diet.

It's such a wide umbrella term for so many bowel disturbances of unknown origin that it's difficult to find a cure for IBS. Since there is no damage in the gut, there is unlikely to be any blood in the stools, nor will there normally be any weight loss or night time diarrhoea which would suggest a more serious complaint like Crohn's disease or ulcerative colitis. Both complaints deserve a trip to the doctor. IBS, on the other hand, is actually quite a minor complaint as far as the doctor is concerned, but millions of sufferers think otherwise.

The most widely held theory is that it is a stress-related

psychosomatic illness – particularly if it is the constipated variety. If you're one of the thousands who suffer from constant diarrhoea, it could be an intolerance to a certain type of food and you'd have to do an elimination diet to see what was causing it. This involves cutting out all or most of the foods you generally eat for one to three weeks. If the condition improves, gradually reintroduce the foods you've eliminated one by one to see if they affect you. A word of warning: you'll feel terrible at first, not least because you'll be depriving yourself of all your favourite foods, but by the end of the first week you should see results. If, however, nothing has come to light after three weeks, give up. In any case, you should only do this under a doctor's supervision to make sure you're not going to jump to the wrong conclusions.

In many cases it could just be that the muscles of the gut are contracting too much or too little. If you're an IBS sufferer and you find that your urinate a lot, this might be a sign of muscle spasms which are triggered by stress. Or if you can date your IBS back to when you had food poisoning, a course of antibiotics or a hysterectomy, you might have an unhealthy menagerie of bacteria and yeasts playing havoc with your gut flora in your intestine. They will have lodged themselves there when the body was vulnerable and a perfect breeding ground, but are harmless enough even though they will certainly let your bowel know that they're there.

Fighting unhealthy gut flora takes an army of 'good bacteria', but unless you know what the bad stuff is made of, you won't know which regiment to call in. Live yoghurt is your best bet since it contains one of the most important bacteria in the gut, lactobacillus. To make sure that the yoghurt you use really is live, add a spoonful to some warm milk which has been boiled and then cooled. Keep it warm in a vacuum flask for six to eight hours and if it hasn't turned to yoghurt in that time, the original spoonful wasn't live in the first place.

Dr Heaton, who was in charge of the Bristol study, has been interested in bowels for some time. In the eighties he was particularly curious as to why so few attempts had been made to evaluate the effects of fibre on irritable bowel syndrome, considering how many people suffered from it. At that time there were just three reports on bran and the evidence emerging from them was far from conclusive. So Dr Heaton took the decision to review the benefits himself on patients with diverticular disease, the condition in which pouches protrude from the colon. Two out of three of his studies showed that bran had a beneficial effect, but that left him – as a scientist – keen to discover why the other didn't. To date he hasn't found the answer, but he concluded that bran *is* important in the treatment of constipation and that if this is one of the symptoms of the patient's diverticular disease then it should be recommended as a treatment. If, however, it isn't, then he suggested that other foods high in fibre like wholemeal bread and cereals, should be introduced into the diet.

A New York doctor, Dr Leo Galland, found that irritable bowel syndrome could be caused by an intestinal parasite which is picked up from contaminated drinking water. Antibiotics will kill it, but according to physiologist Gordon Leitch at Atlanta's Morehouse School of Medicine, cellulose, the insoluble fibre in corn and wheatbran, can destroy the parasite without giving you the side effects of headaches and depression which antibiotics can induce.

A 1992 study in Aberdeen decided that fibre did relieve IBS, but only in the form of cooked bran cereals like All-Bran and Bran Flakes. Seventy-two patients were asked to record their normal diet over six months and to note the changes when extra fibre was introduced. People in Scotland tend to have a particularly low intake of fruit and vegetables, and their diet sheets showed that the average daily fibre intake of the IBS patients was extremely low mainly because of this. Of the group, 20 had reasonable fibre intake, and of these five men and five women were eating All-Bran or Bran Flakes at some time during the week; two men and three women ate muesli for breakfast but, interestingly, the few who ate raw bran on their food were getting much less of a fibre boost than the breakfast cereal eaters. The others were getting their fibre from baked beans or other pulses and all those with a sufficient fibre rating were eating potatoes and wholemeal bread.

Almost no fruit at all appeared on the diet records and this, according to the Ministry of Agriculture, Fisheries and Foods, is due to price and lack of availability. A high-fibre diet was recommended for the rest of the test group, but when they were asked to note down what they were buying, much of their fibre was coming from relatively poor sources like white bread, cakes, pies and chocolate biscuits. Most of the fibre they were getting was coming from their evening meal, and, as it amounted to well under the recommended level, the study concluded that patients with IBS should be told to eat a cereal such as All-Bran and wholemeal bread for breakfast, which seems to be the easiest meal to pack with fibre.

DIVERTICULAR DISEASE

Diverticular disease is extremely common in this country and comes under the irritable bowel syndrome umbrella. Small pouches are formed through the wall of the colon by pushing and straining and characterise the most common disease of the large intestine. It is found in one in ten people over the age of 40, and one in three over 60. This, Dr Denis Burkitt discovered, was the most rare of Western diseases to be found in the Third World. In fact, the only cases of it he found were among the top social strata in Africa and Asia.

HIATUS HERNIA AND VARICOSE VEINS

Dr Burkitt also noticed that both hiatus hernia – the condition which is characterised by the top of the stomach protruding into the thoracic cavity – and varicose veins are rare in the Third World. In his studies, he found that 44% of American women between 30 and 50 suffered from varicose veins, while in Africa and India the figure was 5% of the whole population. In India, that 5% was mainly made up of trishaw riders whose pedalling under extreme pressure gave them more than just bad veins to deal with.

While varicose veins are easy to spot, it's not so simple with a hiatus hernia. Both are caused by straining and irregular bowel movements, but nausea and indigestion are more often the first signs of a hiatus hernia. If you have any of these symptoms, get your doctor to check it out.

HAEMORRHOIDS

Piles, or haemorrhoids, are the dilation of the veins in or around the anus and can be itchy and painful and can bleed. It's a very common problem in the West and can affect pregnant women and people who have constipation or diarrhoea. A warm bath and suppositories provide quick relief, and a high-fibre diet will sort out the constipation which could have caused them. Piles are almost unheard of in Asia and Africa.

DIABETES

Asian people in particular are prone to diabetes, having a habit of changing their diet when they become wealthier or emigrate to the West. Dr Burkitt found that the people of Nauru in the Pacific have increased their record of diabetes by 40% since the discovery of phosphates there. They've become one of the wealthiest populations in the world in just a few decades, and their adoption of Western habits including the importing of Western foods and a more leisurely lifestyle have been their downfall. It's not just diabetes which has struck them, they have recently reported the emergence of appendicitis, and experts predict that it won't be long before they start to suffer from coronary heart disease, gallstones, hiatus hernia and diverticular disease.

OBESITY

Half the population in America and Western Europe are over-weight, which, Dr Burkitt noticed, was rarely a problem in tribal African communities. Weight seemed to remain stable after puberty, and even fell during middle age whereas it rises in all Western communities. Cancers of the breast, uterus and colon are more likely to develop in obese people.

To quash any theory that the incidence or otherwise of these diseases might have more to do with genetics than affluent diet, Dr Burkitt, as well as a host of other international experts, noticed that they were rare among blacks living in Africa but equally likely to affect black and white people in America. The Japanese, like the Asians, also began to change their eating habits and suffer our diseases once they moved to the West.

CHOLESTEROL

Since Dr Burkitt's work was published, it has been confirmed that fibre also reduces the levels of cholesterol in the blood, the main cause of heart disease particularly in middle-aged men. While insoluble fibre such as the skin, peel and husks of fruit, vegetables and wholegrain products is important in the prevention of colon cancer, it's mainly the water-soluble fibre of beans, oat products and barley which reduces cholesterol.

A concerted effort in America to encourage the general public to find out their cholesterol levels has been extremely successful. The 'Know Your Number' campaign has resulted in most Americans not just being aware of their level, but doing something about it, too. This has not happened in this country, and with two out of three Britons running an increased risk of heart disease because of their high cholesterol levels, can we afford to remain so ignorant? By eating the right low-fat, high-fibre diet we can reduce cholesterol by 30%, which equates to a 60% lower risk of suffering from heart disease.

THE ALARM BELLS

If you recognise any of the following, you should check your cholesterol level as soon as possible. Also, if you smoke, have high blood pressure or are more than 20% overweight, get yourself tested.

- If you have a history of heart disease in your close family
- If your parents, brother or sister has a high cholesterol level
- If you are diabetic
- If you have a whitish ring around the iris in your eye
- If there are hard lumps on the back of your hands or you have enlarged or lumpy Achilles tendons
- If you have yellow patches around your eyelids

Many people have high cholesterol levels without any of the last four symptoms, in which case their bodies are not telling them that they are in danger. One in 500 people inherits a predisposition to high cholesterol which is called familial hypercholesterolaemia (FH) and is just plain bad luck. Since they've had it from birth it will have had more time to do its worst, and they are more likely to suffer from heart disease than the rest of us. A rogue gene makes their bodies less efficient at getting rid of excess cholesterol but a high-fibre, low-fat diet, with olive oil replacing butter, will still reduce the risk of heart disease.

The Department of Health, the Coronary Prevention Group, the Family Heart Association and the British Heart Foundation all believe that we should only get our levels tested in a medical environment where proper advice and, if necessary, treatment can be given immediately.

DIET WATCH

If you have high cholesterol, make sure the following foods are not dominating your diet:

Liver, kidneys, liver paté, shrimps, prawns, fish roe, egg yolks

Soluble fibre (beans, oats, barley) and vitamins A, C and E will reduce cholesterol levels so *do* eat:

Cereals with oat bran, vegetarian dishes with pulses, chickpeas and lentils, fruit (including berries) and yellow and green vegetables

CANCER INHIBITORS

These are thought to include: fibre, beta carotene (found in carrots, cress, spinach, broccoli, tomatoes, mangoes, melons, apricots, peaches and oranges), vitamin E (found in peanuts, soya, corn, safflower and sunflower oils, wheatgerm and cereal grains) and selenium (found in root vegetables).

Wheatbran has been isolated as being of particular significance in the prevention of cancer – especially breast and colon cancer. Study after study shows how fibre acts like a Pacman, gobbling up the potential carcinogens and expelling them in the faeces. Wheatbran fibre has a particular function in preventing the reabsorption of oestrogens, the hormones which can be responsible for breast cancer. These normally circulate within the system, being reabsorbed into the bloodstream and into the liver before being sent on their way again and being dismantled by bacteria in the process. But wheatbran fibre has the opposite effect of a high-fat diet in that it eats up the baddies in the bacteria before they can interact with the oestrogen. Never has All-Bran had such a macho image . . .

Beta carotene is a pigment in certain vegetables and fruits which is made more available when cooked and if vegetables are minced rather than sliced. We eat far too little beta carotene, so we should make sure that we get at least two servings of vegetables a day. The proponents of the Mediterranean diet, who made eating healthily a joy with the news that a cornucopia of delicious foods and olive oils would save our hearts and reduce the risk of cancer, suggest five servings of fruit and vegetables a day. As a nation we're not good at eating our greens, and the thought of mounds of swede and turnip aren't too inspiring. But try looking to Italy, Provence and Greece for your ideas about what to do with a courgette. When you're talking about a whole platter of roasted vegetables for dinner, or grilled peppers marinated in garlic and olive oil with tuna for lunch, then it's no hardship to think about five servings a day. And before you wonder who of all these experts has got it right, notice how they all say the same thing: lots of fibre from your fruit, veg and cereals, olive oil rather than butter, keep your meat intake low and cut the fat off first. Dairy products are dubious because of their fat content, so use low-fat yoghurt, skimmed milk, and fromage frais instead of cream. The message is unequivocal – a low-fat, high-fibre diet will do wonders. It's up to you how you cook these foods, but take a tip from the Mediterraneans and I promise your life will change.

SIX

THE WHOLE STORY

Take a look around the health and diet shelves of any major bookshop and you can't fail to notice how the interest levels in a holistic approach to eating and living have risen massively in the last few years. We've taken a few thousand years to catch on to the fact that food is a natural medicine, and one which if eaten in the right environment and state of mind is the key to lifelong health and happiness. The fact that we decided to ignore the advice of the Chinese, Indians and the Mediterraneans who've been quite happy with their diet since the beginning of time is probably due to centuries of arrogance and imperialism. Now, after the excesses of the eighties and with the shame-faced look at our lifestyles that a recession can enforce, it's time to think again.

The good news is that the overwhelming message is to *eat*. Many of us will have never learnt to cook, existing instead on convenience foods and take-aways. While some of these are nutritious enough for a reasonably healthy diet, the very action of taking a processed dinner out of a packet and shoving it in a microwave doesn't exactly encourage a healthy attitude towards food. The idea of sitting down to eat it in front of the telly, without even taking it out of its tin foil tray, is a habit which an Italian, Spaniard or Moroccan would find bizarre. Virtually every other country in the world makes time for food; mealtimes are sacred and spent with family and friends, with food itself seen as a gift for loved ones. In Italy, everyone from the most macho of young men to the oldest of grandmothers knows how to whip up the most delicious pasta sauce made with fresh plum tomatoes, basil and extra virgin olive oil. Food, they believe, is sacred and, whatever the circumstances, should never be rushed. If the stomach really is the seat of emotion, as the classical poets described, how better to make it feel good than to feed it with the best that nature has to offer?

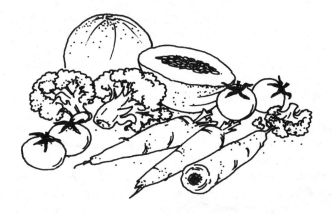

This chapter ties together theories of nutrition, cooking and mental health, and suggests that this more holistic approach could finally blow away the cobwebs of confusion about dieting, digestion and disease. The broader view on fibre as a cleanser or detoxifier might just give you the impetus to kick-start your new eating regime and bin that pattern of self abuse once and for all.

As the profile of the breakfast skipper in Chapter Three illustrated, nutritionists have been busy looking at the psychological difference between people who eat fibre and those who don't. One study, with the snappy little title of 'Dietary Fibre and Personality Factors as Determinants of Stool Output', concludes that it's the extroverts who excrete well, and the less outgoing who might be more 'anally retentive' as it were. Fairly obvious, perhaps, until you find that many people who might *pretend* to be perfectly happy with themselves would give the game away if anyone watched their bathroom habits too closely. The results of this study showed that people who were positive about themselves were more likely to visit their toilets more often, and more effectively.

The whole story lies in the way that the well-adjusted person treats him or herself: if you feed yourself well then you're more likely to be in touch with your body's real needs and to project the image of the well-balanced, happy individual. Buddhists and Hindus alike will say they told us so, but we're finally learning that the external reflects the internal.

Our bodies give us strong messages about what they need to function properly. From the very basic call for liquid if we're not drinking enough to the alarm bells if we've drunk too much, our bodies know exactly what's good and what's bad for them. If we don't hear those warning signals, we could end up with some of the diseases Denis Burkitt highlighted. And if we decide to ignore the warnings, we could also be on the way to sickness. The human body is like a car: fill it with the right fuel and it will run smoothly. If a red light comes on, make sure you fix the problem. But smash the red light and you may have got rid of the warning but the problem won't have gone away. If you're suffering from wind or if your food keeps repeating on you, your body is trying to tell you that you've overworked its digestive system, or that the mix of nutrients you just hap-hazardly chucked down was wrong for it. Ignore it at your peril: too much acid tends to cause these problems, and if you don't balance the scales you might find yourself suffering from skin disorders like eczema and psoriasis, arthritis, rheumatism, and duodenal and peptic ulcers.

Headaches, stomach aches and colds are some of the body's red lights and if we suppress the pain with an aspirin, we're simply smashing those lights. Stress or unhappiness could be the reason for your headache and no amount of paracetamol is going to solve your crisis for you. The body responds immediately to stress and sends out very straightforward messages for you to do something about it. The pituitary gland which is at the base of the brain releases a hormone into the bloodstream which in turn alerts the adrenals (two more glands which are found in the kidneys). The adrenals then send out some more hormones; at the same time the nervous system has picked up on the messages and adrenalin is activated.

Adrenalin can make us jumpy, ratty and unable to sleep, our brains working overtime. This is stress, and if we don't do anything to alleviate the cause, the symptoms certainly won't let us off the hook. Relax. Exercise. Above all, eat. If you take time out of your busiest of days to eat with friends or family, you'll probably find yourself unwinding and laughing about your strange priorities.

The principles of naturopathy – the idea that the body can heal itself – have finally been absorbed by the more enlightened members of the food industry. Luckily, their sales figures can only be helped by the promotion of the idea that products such as fibre can prevent a myriad of life-threatening diseases. Finally, industry and nature are beginning to join forces as our bodies breathe a sigh of relief.

DETOXIFICATION

Detoxing – the natural cleansing of the body – used to be something weird people did on a yoga weekend in the Home Counties but now, with better information about how food works, detoxing is entering the mainstream. The idea is simple – we all need to shut the world out from time to time, switch everything off and relax. But the body doesn't have time to do this if we spend that time drinking alcohol or caffeine and eating chocolate and fried foods as we tend to do when we're on holiday. The body is a machine which occasionally needs to be shut down too. Fasting is one of the best ways of doing this, so that the body has literally nothing to do other than to right some of the wrongs to which it's been subjected. Nutrition expert Professor Arnold Ehret once said, 'Man digs his grave with his knife and fork' and strongly recommended the age-old health habit of fasting. When we're ill, we often lose our appetite, which is the body's way of dealing with the main fight to get better. To eat under those circumstances would be to clog up the natural machinery while it's working overtime. Take a tip from animals and the instinctive way they fast when they need to heal themselves.

I spent one of those wacky weekends in the Home Counties after my brain and body had been screaming at me for some let up in a ridiculously busy routine. No caffeine, lots of water, herbal teas and no food at all for 48 hours left me feeling incredibly refreshed and surprisingly energetic for days afterwards and gave me the impetus to change my eating habits for ever. It's only when you give yourself a breather and realise how much you needed that fast, sleep, or alcohol break that you recognise how abusive your habits have been.

For many people, the idea of having 48 hours to yourself with very few demands for expending any energy is no more than a pipe dream. If such an opportunity were to arise, you're not likely to spend it fasting. But you *can* get rid of your cellulite and get your body working properly while still eating. Food itself can be a detoxifier, and none better than fibre. Short grain brown rice is the staple of a detox diet because it contains a lot of fibre and B vitamins. It is broken down and digested more quickly than the long grain, and its absorbative qualities mean that it literally soaks up the toxins which are playing havoc with your gut. By eating a lot of fruit and vegetables and drinking lots of water you will be spending a lot more time in the toilet than normal, and those toxins won't know what hit them. Once the gut has been cleaned by the fluid and brown rice, the healthy bacteria that should be there can grow and do their job of extracting the goodness from food without any obstacles.

ENEMAS

For those who really want to dive in at the deep end of the health revolution, there's always the enema. It involves the flushing of water into the large bowel, which then allows complete evacuation of any waste in the system. If you're eating a diet rich in fibre, with plenty of anti-oxidants from your fruit and vegetables, you shouldn't have to rely on enemas for keeping your colon so clean that carcinogens don't stand a chance in promoting cancer. But a total clean-out from an enema is like a fast – it gives the overloaded body time to get rid of all the toxins and start again. However, it's *always* a good idea to take an enema under proper medical supervision, and *not* experiment on your own.

In many countries in the East, enemas are seen as the key to inner health. Nepalis, Indians and Chinese have always known that most diseases come from the colon, and that it's a good idea to keep it clean. Now, as with so many Eastern philosophies, enemas have become more popular in the West as we realise that sometimes our bodies need a little help. In the Netherlands, naturopath Jan de Vries designed an apparatus for cleaning the upper bowel and remembers the first time he used it on a patient: 'The treatment involved flushing approximately 30 pints of camomile water through the bowels and we were absolutely astonished at the quantity of waste material consequently disposed of.'

Eastern gurus believe that the enema remains the most effective and gentlest way of caring for the bowels. It can make you feel better, bring relief from hunger pangs and cure head-aches and muscular aches. They claim that it is one of the most important ways for the whole family to treat fever and other upsets. And millions of people in the East agree.

Rather than polluting your system again after an enema, try drinking less traditional and more herbal teas. There are plenty available and, as they don't require milk, they are also better for people watching their weight. We also need fibre to sweep the debris from our system. Water is just as essential, clearing out the toxins and helping just about every organ in our bodies to function normally. Over 60% of the body is made up of water, and it is the loss of this in so many diets which brings about the rapid weight loss in the first couple of weeks.

Naturopaths believe that there are plenty of natural foods which boost the system when it needs it. Seaweed, for example, is rich in iodine which speeds up the metabolism; cayenne and ginger stimulate the digestive tract, purify the blood and encourage the toxins to sweat out through the skin. Too much of either will have an abrasive effect on the stomach wall, but in small amounts they can be extremely beneficial. If you've found that you can't do anything to stop lentils and pulses giving you wind, try adding a little dried or grated root ginger. Garlic is famous for being a purifier and has been used for centuries as a herbal medicine. It is said to lower blood pressure and ease mucus conditions as well as bronchitis. Parsley is garlic's natural antidote in terms of cleaning the breath, but once garlic is being regularly absorbed into your diet you'll find that it leaves no smell at all.

Beetroot is supposed to be a tonic for the liver. After a bout of excessive drinking try eating some beetroot. It has a propensity to turn urine red for a while, but this is perfectly normal.

If you're going to stop abusing your body by detoxing, changing your diet and having the occasional supervised enema, why not start brushing your skin every morning too? This is one of the most invigorating ways to start your day and stimulates the circulation which is – among other things – responsible for banishing cellulite. Your skin will be much softer, and if you rub some oil on after your brush and shower it will look smoother too. Get a bristle brush from a chemist or the Body Shop, and first thing every morning brush your skin while it's dry, starting at the feet and working your way up each leg followed by your back, buttocks, stomach and chest before finishing by brushing down the back of your neck. Always brush towards your heart, and avoid irritated areas or abrasions. This seemingly masochistic ritual is something that yoga teachers highly recommend. It unclogs the pores, clearing all the dead cells, and allows the skin to breathe properly. It can eliminate uric acid which causes cystitis, as well as a host of other toxins, taking a heavy burden off your kidneys and liver.

Dry skin brushing also stimulates the lymphatic system which collects toxins from the cells and takes them to the lymph glands to be processed and neutralised. Swollen glands when we're ill are a result of the cellular debris the lymphatic system has dumped in the lymph nodes. As it throws itself into a full-scale war against the infection in another part of the body, a lot of extra rubbish has to be removed from the battle site and stored in these glands. Even though the glands work overtime to neutralise the germs there's bound to be a bit of congestion and this is evident in the swelling. The largest collection of lymph glands is near the heart, and dry skin brushing, apart from stimulating the blood circulation, will also accelerate the flow of the lymph system, cleaning it out much more thoroughly.

Following a detox diet for a week should actually be no different from your normal diet if you've taken on board the

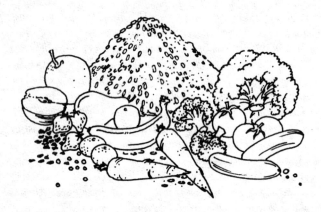

advice here in *Fibrenetics*. Fibre from cereals, fruit and vegetables will clear out the system every day. However, some people need to follow eating plans if they are to do a detox, or a weight-loss regime. Counting calories discourages a love of food and casts it as the enemy in a weight war, whereas after reading this book you should be able to wander around the supermarket and know just what each food group can do for you. If you're feeling tired and need a refreshing detox you'll automatically stock up on raw vegetables, while if you've overdone the drinking you'll instinctively go for beetroot. The brown rice and cereals shelf will say FIBRE to you, and if you're a little constipated you'll add a few extra packets to your trolley. Breakfast cereals will become a must in the same way fruit and vegetables will. Do buy the detox books for the recipes, and find out how marinated kebabs, chicory and fennel in coriander dressing and kiwi and ginger salad will make any detox a joy. But also learn to rely on your new love of food: be inventive and stun your friends with endless ways of making salads, cereals, vegetables and lentils interesting.

The big change is in attitude. When you feel so much better, your eyes will shine, you'll be full of energy and you'll have fallen in love with the best food in the world after years of deprivation and suspicion. Fast and fatty food will be the last thing on your mind. It's not even a matter of weaning yourself off the bad stuff and on to the healthy, but more a sudden recognition that this is what you've been looking for all this time – a way of eating great food, losing weight and keeping it off, looking and feeling better and having the energy to do all those things you always wanted to do with your life. Food cannot be the enemy any more: it's nature's best present and it can bring out the best in every single one of us. So eat, drink and be merry, and you're much more likely to live to a ripe old age.

THE BEANFEAST

The recipes in this final section of the book come from British restaurants which have given the tarnished image of our national cuisine a respray. Rising to the challenge of cooking healthier foods, they've proved that they can do anything with a lentil, and that low fat certainly doesn't have to mean low taste. If you think that eating out or cooking great food at home is going to be impossible on your low-fat/high-fibre regime, take another look at what's happening in the world of food.

THE PEAT INN

By Cupar, Fife. Tel. 033484 206

David Wilson says that his food reflects the region. It may be difficult to find a supermarket in Scotland but at the Peat Inn at least, its broths and lentils are as popular today as they've always been . . .

CHICKEN IN A POT WITH VEGETABLES, FRESH HERBS AND PULSES

Serves four

1 fresh chicken about $3\frac{1}{2}$–4lb (1.5–1.8kg)

Ingredients for poaching liquid

4 pt (approx $2\frac{1}{4}$ litres) chicken stock

2 small onions, peeled, each studded with a bay leaf and two cloves

2 cloves garlic, peeled

1 white of leek tied with bunch of fresh herbs (chervil or parsley, tarragon, thyme)

4 black peppercorns

Ingredients for finished dish

8 pieces celery (peeled) about $1\frac{1}{2}$in. (4cm) long

8 pieces white of leek about 1in. ($2\frac{1}{2}$cm) long

8 baby carrots or carrots turned to about 2in (5cm) long

8 small turned potatoes

4 oz (100g) broth mix (soak overnight in cold water)

1 tbsp chopped chervil or flat parsley

1 tbsp chopped chives

salt and pepper

Fill a large pot with chicken stock, add ingredients for poaching liquid, bring to boil and simmer for approx. 25 minutes.

Add whole chicken, bring back to boil and simmer for a further 20 minutes.

Remove chicken, remove skin, strain poaching liquid discarding vegetables etc., and remove fat from surface of poaching liquid with kitchen paper. Return liquid and chicken to clean pot.

Add ingredients for finished dish, bring back to boil, then simmer for about 10 minutes.

Remove chicken, cut into 8 pieces and arrange in 4 warm soup plates. Remove vegetables from cooking liquid with slotted spoon and divide among 4 plates. Season stock to taste, then ladle stock, with the broth mix, over chicken. Finish by sprinkling chopped chervil and chives over dish. Serve immediately.

SOHO SOHO

Frith St, London W1. Tel. 071 494 3491

Chef Tony Howarth cooks quintessential Mediterranean diet food which knocks on the head any idea that healthy food has to be dull. His fibre-packed rolls alone are an inspiration to anyone who loves the smell of freshly baked bread mixed with olives, tomatoes or mushrooms

SALADE D'ASPERGES ET LENTILLES

Serves six

12 oz (350g) cooked asparagus

2oz (50g) carrots, peeled and sliced into ribbons

2oz (50g) courgettes, sliced into ribbons

1oz (25g) sliced red onion

1oz (25g) oyster mushrooms

A selection of lettuce (the best are: spider, frisée, radicchio, gem, rocket. Don't use round lettuce)

Lentil vinaigrette

3oz (75g) cooked puy lentils

1 tbsp Dijon mustard

3 tbsp sherry vinegar

2 tsp (10ml) walnut oil

2 chopped shallots

1 clove garlic crushed

Salt and pepper

Cut the heads off the asparagus 1 inch from the top and cut the rest of the stalk into strips on the bias.

Grill vegetables on a char grill. For best results without a char grill, heat a thick-bottomed frying pan until dry and very hot.

Without using oil, lay the strips of vegetable in the pan until they colour.

Wash all the lettuce and pull apart.

Mix the ingredients for the lentil vinaigrette together.

Toss all the ingredients in a large bowl so as not to crush the salad. Arrange on 6 plates (try to keep some height to the salad).

PAIN À LA TOMATE SECHÉE

Makes two loaves

1 garlic clove, crushed	236ml (8fl.oz) water
4 tbsp chopped onion	125g (5oz) chopped sun dried tomatoes
1 tbsp sun dried tomato oil	
20g ($\frac{3}{4}$–1oz) fresh yeast (mix with 57ml (2fl.oz) tepid water to start fermentation)	500g (1lb) unbleached flour
	Pinch of salt

Sauté the garlic, onion and tomato oil together.

Depending on the flour used you may need to reduce the water a little. Put all the ingredients in a mixer and beat for 2 minutes with the dough hook. Alternatively, it can be brought together by hand and worked until the elasticity has been brought out i.e. when pressed the dough springs back.

Put in an oiled bowl, cover with a damp cloth and let it double in size.

Knead again and make into 2 loaves.

Rub with some olive oil and let them prove. When they have risen bake them in the oven at 400°F/200°C/Gas 6 for 30 minutes, spraying with water 3 times in the first 10 minutes.

PAIN AUX OLIVES

20g ($\frac{3}{4}$–1oz) fresh yeast (mix with
150ml ($\frac{1}{4}$pt) tepid water to start
fermentation)
60ml (4 tbsp) olive oil

30 chopped green stoned olives
30 chopped black stoned olives
500g (1lb) flour
8g ($\frac{1}{4}$oz) salt

Follow the instructions for making the dough from the previous recipe for tomato bread.

PAIN AUX CHAMPIGNONS

2 tbsp olive oil
125g (5oz) field mushrooms, sliced
25g (1oz) dried cèpe mushrooms
(infused in 330ml ($\frac{1}{2}$ pt) boiling
water until tepid)
60ml (4tbsp) olive oil

10g ($\frac{1}{3}$ oz) fresh yeast
500g (1lb) flour
1 tbsp salt
1 tbsp minced garlic

Sauté the field mushrooms with 2 tablespoons of olive oil and allow to cool.

Follow the instructions for making the dough from the recipe for tomato bread opposite.

DELL'UGO

56 Frith St, London W1. Tel. 071 734 8300

Antony Worral-Thompson is so dedicated to the pleasures of the Mediterranean that he called his restaurant after a type of olive oil.

A SALAD OF LENTILS WITH SPINACH AND LIME

$\frac{1}{2}$ lb (225g) puy lentils
Vegetable stock, to cover
1 cup* finely diced onions
$2\frac{1}{2}$ fl.oz (75ml) virgin olive oil
3 cloves garlic, peeled and finely chopped

1 chilli, seeded and finely diced
$\frac{1}{4}$ cup chopped fresh coriander
10 oz (300g) cooked spinach, finely chopped
2 potatoes, peeled and cubed
Salt and ground black pepper
$2\frac{1}{2}$ fl.oz (75ml) fresh lime juice

Cook lentils in stock for about 20 minutes then drain, retaining cooking liquor.

Meanwhile, brown the onions in oil until golden. Add garlic, chilli and coriander with the spinach and pan fry for 5–6 minutes.

Add potatoes and lentil cooking liquid to cover. Season.

After 25 minutes, add lentils and simmer for a further 15 minutes or until thick and soupy.

Add lime juice; season to taste. Serve warm or cold.

*1 cup = 10 fl.oz (300 ml)

THE ARTS THEATRE CAFE

Gt Newport St, Leicester Square, London WC1.
Tel. 071 497 8014

Phil Owens has incorporated the low-fat/high-fibre habit into Sicilian cooking, and come up with recipes which cured his arthritis and helped him shed two stone. Try his delicious pasta recipe:

PASTA WITH CHICK-PEAS, SAVOY CABBAGE PANCETTA AND PARMESAN

9 oz (250g) chick-peas
14 oz (400g) tinned tomatoes
3 cloves of garlic (1$\frac{1}{2}$ for each stage)
10 oz (300g) penne
2 anchovy fillets
2 tbsp olive oil

4 oz (100g) pancetta
$\frac{1}{2}$ savoy cabbage, shredded
Salt and pepper
$\frac{1}{2}$ tsp red chilli flakes, to taste
3 oz (75g) parmesan, freshly grated

Soak chick-peas for 24 hours and cook in abundant water for about 2 hours with $\frac{1}{2}$ teaspoon of bicarbonate of soda to tenderise.

Make your own tomato paste (it is useful to make extra as it keeps well in the fridge with a layer of olive oil over the top of the jar). Empty tin of tomatoes into a saucepan, add garlic and reduce over a low heat till a thick paste is formed. Pass through a food mill.

Cook pasta according to instructions.

While it is cooking fry remaining garlic and anchovy in olive oil till anchovy melts. Add pancetta, fry for 2 minutes and add savoy cabbage. Season with salt, pepper and chilli flakes. Cook till it wilts and add tomato paste and cooked chick-peas. Toss with the pasta and add tablespoon of pasta water, taste for seasoning.

Place in warmed bowls and sprinkle with parmesan.

LE MERIDIEN

Piccadilly, London W1. Tel. 071 734 8000

David Chambers reckons that while low fat lends itself perfectly to haute cuisine, there's not a lot you can do with fibre. Except perhaps the following . . .

ST PIERRE AUX LENTILLES DU PUY

(John Dory on a bed of green lentils)

1 oz (30g) carrot, $\frac{1}{4}$cm dice
1 oz (30g) onion
$\frac{1}{2}$ oz (15g) celeriac
$\frac{1}{2}$ oz (15g) leek
$\frac{3}{4}$ oz (20g) smoked back bacon (very fine julienne)
9 oz (250g) green lentils

1 pt (600ml) fish stock
Salt and pepper
Bouquet garni
$\frac{1}{3}$ pt (200ml) Newcastle brown ale
$\frac{1}{4}$ oz (10g) shallots
7 oz (200g) unsalted butter
4 fillets of John Dory, approx. 5–6oz (150g) each
Diced tomato

Sweat the carrot, onion, celeriac, leek and bacon in a little butter, then add lentils and continue to sweat.

Add $\frac{3}{4}$ pint fish stock, a little salt and pepper and the bouquet garni. Simmer for 1 $\frac{1}{2}$ hours, stirring occasionally.

Reduce the brown ale and shallots almost to a glaze, add the remaining fish stock and reduce again. Add in the butter very slowly, whisking continuously. Check the seasoning.

Sauté the fish in a little butter to achieve a light golden colour. Remove from pan and keep warm.

Arrange 5 small spoons of lentils around the plate to form a star pattern. Place the fish on the lentils half covering them. Put the diced tomato in between each piece of fish.

Pass the sauce and pour around the plate. Garnish with a little fresh chervil.

FLAN DE LENTILLES DU PUY AUX CHOUX VERT

(Savoy cabbage and lentil flan)
Serves six

1 large savoy cabbage

Lentilles

1 oz (30g) onions, diced

1 oz (30g) carrots, diced

½ oz (15g) leeks, diced

½ oz (15g) celeriac, diced

2 oz (50g) butter

¾ oz (20g) bacon (finely chopped) – optional

7 oz (200g) baby green lentils

1 pt (600ml) chicken stock

1 bouquet garni

Salt and pepper

Tomato coulis

2 lb (800g) tomatoes

1 oz (25g) chopped shallot or onion

1 oz (25g) butter, margarine or oil

Salt and pepper

Lentilles

Sweat the diced vegetables in butter.

Add bacon and cook for a few minutes. Add lentils and continue to cook, stirring for a further minute.

Add the chicken stock, bouquet garni and salt and pepper to taste. Bring to the boil.

Cover and cook slowly for 1 hour. The lentils should remain slightly moist.

Tomato coulis

Remove the stalks from the tomatoes. Plunge them into boiling water for 5–6 seconds. Refresh immediately.

Remove the skins, cut in half crosswise, and remove the seeds.

Roughly chop the tomato flesh.

Meanwhile cook the chopped onion or shallot in butter without colouring.

Add the tomatoes and season.

Simmer gently until cooked.

Blend tomatoes in a liquidiser, adding a small amount of chicken stock if required, then pass through sieve and keep warm.

Cabbage

Remove discoloured leaves. Choose 10 best large leaves and blanch in boiling salted water for 5 minutes until limp, then refresh in iced water and dry out on clean towel.

With a sharp knife remove large part of centre stalk.

The remainder of the cabbage should be finely shredded, boiled for 10 minutes, refreshed in iced water, thoroughly squeezed dry and added to cooked lentils.

Taking a 8 inch (20 cm) flan ring, place on a non-stick baking tray and butter both well.

Line the mould (flan ring) with the cabbage leaves leaving a good overlap and double layer on the bottom. Then season with salt and pepper.

Fill the flan with lentils to the edge of mould, fold over leaves adding some more on top, then cover with well-buttered tin foil and cook in a moderate oven for 1 hour.

Remove ring and portion into wedges. Sauce plates with tomato coulis and place flan on top. Decorate with fresh chervil.

THE GIBBON BRIDGE HOTEL

Chipping, Lancs. Tel. 0995 61456

Janet Simpson started her career in catering as a baker, and took her fibre ideas with her to set up the Gibbon Bridge. The food's a bit fancier these days, but the principles of low fat and high fibre have had nowt taken out.

CARROT AND CAULIFLOWER SOUP

1 large onion
2pt (1 litre) vegetable stock
1lb (500g) carrots

1lb (500g) cauliflower
1 large potato

Sweat the onions in some of the stock until transparent and soft.

Chop all vegetables into similar sized pieces, place in pan with onions and remainder of stock. Season and add a dash of Worcestershire sauce. Boil until tender, drain and reserve liquor.

Liquidize vegetables, recombine and pass through a sieve till smooth.

Let down soup with skimmed milk. Reheat and serve with a spoonful of Greek yoghurt and herbs to garnish.

FILLET OF SMOKED TROUT WITH A 'BONFIRE' OF SALAD LEAVES

Wash and gently 'rip' apart a variety of salad leaves, both red and green. Use as many varieties of colour and shape as possible to achieve the best effect. Ensure most of the water is removed then place combined leaves in a 'bonfire' shape to one side of the plate. Lightly coat with a white wine vinaigrette.

Place fillet of smoked trout beside the leaves and garnish with a decorative piece of lemon. Serve as a starter.

SUMMER PUDDING

2lb (1kg) mixed fruit from:
strawberries, raspberries,
redcurrants, blackcurrants,
blackberries

10 oz (300g) desert apples,
peeled, cored and chopped
roughly

8 oz (225g) sugar
$\frac{1}{4}$ pt (150ml) water
White bread, sliced

Place all the fruits, sugar and water in a pan and bring to the boil. Remove from the heat and drain but reserve the juices.

Allow fruits to cool while preparing the mould.

Line a pudding basin or loaf tin with cling film then cut crusts off slices of white bread. Dip the bread in the fruit juice and line the bowl/tin so that the bottom and all sides are covered. Cut a piece of bread to fit the top as a lid.

Fill the breaded container with the fruits and pack well in. Add juice and cover with 'bread lid'. Weight down and chill in the refrigerator overnight.

THE UNION CLUB

Greek St, London W 1.

Carolyn Dawson is the chef at London's funkiest new members' club and if that sounds élitist, well, it is. The food, however, isn't.

WHOLEMEAL LINGUINE WITH SPINACH, PEAS, WALNUTS, FROMAGE FRAIS AND PARMESAN

Serves four

1lb (500g) fresh wholemeal
linguine
11fl.oz (350ml) fromage frais
$\frac{1}{4}$ tsp garlic, crushed
2 bunches of washed and picked
spinach

1 cup* fresh peas, blanched
$\frac{1}{2}$ cup walnuts
8 oz (225g) parmesan, freshly
grated

Put linguine into boiling water and cook for 3–5 minutes.

Heat fromage frais in a saucepan with the garlic and reduce until a little thicker. Add chopped spinach, peas and walnuts and season with salt and pepper.

Bring to the boil and add drained linguine.

Serve with freshly grated parmesan on top.

* 1 cup = 10fl.oz (300ml)

MULTIGRAIN BREAD

Makes two loaves

500ml (16fl.oz) water
40g (1½ oz) yeast
500g (1lb) white flour
425g (15 oz) wholemeal flour
½ tbsp golden syrup

20g (¾ oz) salt
150ml (5fl.oz) oil
¼ cup* each of rolled oats, rye, millet and sesame seeds

Warm up a little of the water and dissolve yeast in it with a teaspoon of sugar. When foaming add to all the other ingredients and the rest of the water.

Knead the dough until smooth. Cover and prove until double in size. Knead again and form into 2 loaf shapes. Prove for a further 15–20 minutes and bake at 450°F/230°C/Gas 8 until golden brown.

*1 cup = 10 fl.oz (300 ml)

POTATO, WATERCRESS AND BASIL SOUP

Serves six

3 diced potatoes (unpeeled)
3 cups* chicken stock (use water if vegetarian)
4 tbsp unsalted butter
2 leeks, washed
1 small onion, diced

½ cup (tightly packed) watercress leaves
¼ cup fresh basil leaves
1 cup (½ pt) of milk
salt and freshly ground black pepper

Boil potatoes until tender in stock. Melt butter in pan and sweat diced leeks and onion until soft. Add watercress and stir until wilted down. Process all together in food processor until smooth, adding the basil last.

Strain and add milk, salt and pepper to taste and a dash of freshly grated nutmeg if desired.

* 1 cup = 10fl.oz (300ml)

LENTIL SALAD WITH CURLY ENDIVE

Serves four

1 curly endive
2 cups* cooked lentils
1 cooked beetroot, finely diced
$\frac{1}{4}$ cup toasted pinenuts
1 tbsp chopped parsley
$\frac{1}{2}$ white onion, finely diced
4 rashers lean bacon, finely diced and fried crisp (optional for vegetarians)

$\frac{1}{4}$ cup (2 $\frac{1}{2}$fl.oz) vinaigrette (tbsp vinegar, 1 tsp Dijon mustard, $\frac{1}{4}$ tsp crushed garlic, $\frac{1}{4}$ cup (2 $\frac{1}{2}$fl.oz) olive oil, salt and pepper to taste)

Wash curly endive and drain. Mix all ingredients except endive and dress with some of the vinaigrette. Spread lentils on to a plate and top with endive dressed in the rest of the vinaigrette.

*1 cup = 10 fl.oz (300 ml)

HYATT CUISINE NATURELLE

Here are a number of recipes from the innovative cuisine naturelle range developed by the Hyatt hotel chain (see p. 102)

TURKEY CARBONARA

Serves four

1 lb whole wheat linguini	4 oz green peas
6 oz carbonara sauce (see recipe)	3 tbsp fresh herbs
4 oz lean bacon, cut in strips	2 tbsp vegetable seasoning
olive oil	ground black pepper, to taste
4 shallots, minced	1 tbsp fresh basil, chopped
4 cloves garlic, minced	

Cook pasta, drain, reserve for later use.

Prepare carbonara sauce (see below).

Cook bacon strips, having removed all fat first.

Lightly coat large sauté pan with olive oil. Heat, and add bacon strips, then shallots and garlic. Begin to cook over low heat.

Add pasta, peas, and fresh herbs and sauté quickly. Then add carbonara sauce. Bring to boil and season with a little salt and black pepper.

Pour onto serving plate; garnish with chopped fresh basil. Serve immediately.

Sauce

$\frac{1}{2}$ oz corn oil margarine	ground black pepper, to taste
1 oz flour	garlic herb seasoning to taste
10 oz skimmed milk	1 oz parmesan cheese
1 $\frac{1}{2}$ fl.oz white wine	
2 oz skimmed ricotta cheese	

Preheat margarine and stir in flour slowly. Heat for 1 or 2 minutes, stirring occasionally. Add skimmed milk, then wine, then ricotta and seasonings. Stir. Bring to boil, simmering slowly till thickened. Add parmesan and lightly simmer for 1 minute.

MARINATED PORK TENDERLOIN

Serves four

1$\frac{1}{2}$lb pork tenderloin	$\frac{1}{2}$ oz onion
$\frac{1}{2}$ oz low sodium soy sauce	1 shitake mushroom
2 tsp ginger	fresh herbs to taste
8 oz red wine	1 lb whole wheat fettucine
1 oz mustard	1 tsp garlic seasoning
1 tbsp basil, chopped	12 oz tomato sauce (see recipe on p. 169)
2 oz lemon juice	
1 oz carrot, quartered	8 tbsp fresh basil, chopped
$\frac{1}{2}$ oz green beans	12 oz black bean relish (see recipe on p. 172)
1 oz fennel	

Trim all fat from pork tenderloin. Mix soy, ginger, wine, mustard, basil and lemon juice for marinade. Marinade pork overnight.

Bring water to a boil and add vegetables. Cook for one minute then drain.

Sear the marinated pork in pan lightly coated with vegetable oil. Put in oven and cook at 375°F/190°C for 10 minutes. Take pork out of pan, and in same pan sauté the blanched vegetables with fresh herbs and seasoning. Add pork to vegetable sauté. Add 2 tbsp of pork marinade and cook for 1 minute.

Prepare fettucine according to directions.

In a separate pan, mix together the tomato sauce and fresh basil. Add prepared pasta and cook lightly. Pour onto plate. Cut pork into 1 inch slices. Spoon pork and vegetable mixture into middle of plate. Spoon black bean relish to side. `

TOMATO SAUCE

Serves four

1 tbsp olive oil	$\frac{1}{2}$ tbsp fresh basil
small white onion	8 oz tomatoes, skinned and seeded
$\frac{1}{2}$ oz garlic	
1 tbsp shallots	8 oz peeled tomatoes (canned)
$\frac{1}{2}$ tbsp thyme	salt to taste
pinch rosemary	pinch white pepper
$\frac{1}{2}$ tbsp oregano	garlic seasoning, to taste

Sauté onions, garlic, shallots and herbs in olive oil in a medium pan till onions are transparent.

Add fresh tomatoes and canned tomatoes. Cook for 5 minutes at full heat, then lower heat, and continue cooking till sauce has reduced to one third (approximately 5–10 minutes).

Add seasoning. Cook for about 1 hour; stirring occasionally. Do not grind or blend, leave chunky.

WHOLE WHEAT PIZZA DOUGH

Serves four

$\frac{1}{3}$ oz yeast

pinch sugar

$2\frac{1}{2}$ oz water

5 oz high gluten flour

12 oz whole wheat flour

$\frac{1}{2}$ tbsp honey

$\frac{1}{2}$ tbsp olive oil

salt to taste

Mix yeast and sugar with warm water in large mixing bowl. Add remaining ingredients. Mix with dough hook on first speed for 8–10 minutes.

Refrigerate dough until needed, then portion out into 4 oz portions.

MEDITERRANEAN GRILLED SANDWICHES

Serves four

1 lb pizza dough (see recipe)

8 slices aubergine

8 slices courgette

8 slices yellow squash

8 each red, yellow, green pepper strips

a pinch of salt and pepper

12 oz chicken strips

4 oz chicken stock

4 oz shredded lettuce

4 oz cuisine herb vinaigrette (see recipe on p. 171)

4 blue corn tortillas

12 oz black bean relish (see recipe on p. 172)

Prepare pizza dough.

Steam all the vegetables except for the lettuce. Lightly coat a frying pan with oil, and heat. Sauté chicken. Add the steamed vegetables, salt and pepper, and chicken stock and quickly sauté.

Roll pizza dough into 10 inch rounds. Grill on very hot flat top for 1 minute and turn. Grill for another minute.

While dough is still warm, top with sautéed vegetables, chicken and shredded lettuce. Drizzle with cuisine herb vinaigrette. Roll up and wrap in a piece of parchment paper.

Meanwhile brush the blue corn tortillas with a very little vegetable oil. Place on hot flat top and grill till crispy. Cut into 6 wedges.

Serve with black bean relish.

CUISINE HERB VINAIGRETTE

Serves ten

2 cups chicken stock
2 cups olive oil
4 cups balsamic vinegar
½ oz corn starch
dash diced fresh garlic
pinch coarse black pepper

fresh thyme, to taste
1 oz fresh parsley, chopped
1 oz fresh basil, chopped
2 tsp fresh oregano, chopped
1 oz chive, chopped

Heat chicken broth. Reduce by one third. Add oil and vinegar. Thicken with corn starch. Simmer for one minute.

Take off heat and cool. Add remaining ingredients and refrigerate for at least an hour.

BLACK BEAN RELISH

Serves four

12 oz cooked black beans	1 tbsp shallots, finely diced
1 oz lime juice	1½ tbsp cilantro, chopped
2½ oz cuisine herb vinaigrette (see recipe on p. 171)	1 tbsp each yellow, red and green pepper, finely diced
1 tsp garlic, finely diced	1 tbsp plum tomatoes, diced

Mix all ingredients together with black beans. Let sit for at least one hour before serving.

BEEF STEW

Serves four

1lb Filet tip of lean beef	4 oz fennel
Marinade (see recipe)	4 oz green beans
2 tbsp garlic seasoning	2 oz chives
2 oz onions, chopped	2 tbsp basil, chopped
½ cup red wine	2 tsp thyme
4 oz carrots	ground black pepper to taste
4 oz courgettes	2 cups beef stock
4 oz tomato	

Trim beef of any fat, and cut into one-inch pieces. Marinade overnight in prepared marinade.

Brush non-stick skillet with a very little cooking oil. Season beef with 1 tbsp garlic seasoning. Sear beef with onions in the hot skillet. Add red wine. Remove beef. Add steamed vegetables to same skillet and season with basil, thyme, remaining 1 tbsp of garlic seasoning and beef stock. Reduce halfway. Add beef back to pan and cook quickly. Serve.

Marinade

4 cups* chicken stock	1 lemon
$1\frac{1}{4}$ cup* white wine	1 lime
1 oz olive oil	1 bay leaf
1 oz fresh herbs	

Heat chicken stock, reduce by one-third. Add wine, olive oil, and herbs. Stir. Squeeze in lemon and lime juice. Simmer for 5 minutes. Chill overnight.

1 US cup = 8 fl.oz (227 ml)

CARROT CAKE

Serves eight

2 cups* wholewheat flour	$1\frac{3}{4}$ cups* grated carrots
$1\frac{1}{2}$ tsp baking powder	$1\frac{1}{2}$ cups* egg whites
$\frac{2}{3}$ tsp cinnamon	$1\frac{1}{2}$ cups* honey
$\frac{1}{4}$ tsp baking soda	Bavarian cream (see recipe on p. 174)
$\frac{1}{8}$ tsp nutmeg	
2 eggs	$\frac{1}{4}$ cup apple juice
1 cup* & 2 tbsp corn oil	mint leaf (optional)

Stir together dry ingredients. Combine eggs and oil. Add dry ingredients to eggs, whip 3 minutes. Add $1\frac{1}{2}$ cups grated carrots, reserving $\frac{1}{4}$ cup for garnish. Whip egg whites and honey till medium firm. Fold into carrot mixture. Pour into round cake pan. Bake for 50 minutes at 350°F/180°C/Gas 4.

Slice cake into 8 wedges. Place a wedge on plate. Mix Bavarian cream with $\frac{1}{4}$ cup grated carrots and apple juice to thin. Drizzle on cake and garnish with mint leaf, if wished.

1 US cup = 8 fl.oz (227 ml)

BAVARIAN CREAM

$\frac{1}{4}$ cup* pure maple sugar	$\frac{1}{4}$ tsp vanilla extract
$\frac{1}{3}$ cup* skimmed ricotta cheese	$\frac{1}{2}$ tsp gelatin
$\frac{1}{3}$ cup* low-fat plain yoghurt	1 tsp water

Mix maple syrup, ricotta cheese, yoghurt, and vanilla in blender. Whip till smooth.

Dissolve gelatin in warm water.

Add a little of the mixture to dissolved gelatin. Slowly mix gelatin into the rest of the mixture. Chill overnight.

1 US cup = 8 fl.oz (227 ml)

CUISINE NATURELLE FRENCH TOAST

Serves four

2 eggs	**8 oz strawberry sauce (see recipe**
8 oz skimmed milk	**on p. 175)**
2 tsp vanilla extract	**4 mint leaves (optional)**
4 vanilla beans, split	
12 slices wholewheat bread	

Whip together eggs, skimmed milk, vanilla, and vanilla beans (for added fresh flavour). Dip bread into liquid mixture, allowing liquid to be absorbed.

Brush a frying pan with a little vegetable oil. Carefully place soaked bread in pan, cooking on both sides until golden brown.

Top French toast with strawberry sauce. Garnish with mint leaves.

STRAWBERRY SAUCE

Serves four

8 oz fresh ripe strawberries

2 oz all fruit (fruit-juice-sweetened) strawberry jam

Purée strawberries until smooth. Add fruit spread and mix well.

Pass through strainer to remove all seeds. Serve.

KELLOGG'S WHEATBRAN RECIPES

Wheatbran is said to be particularly effective in the prevention of cancer – especially of the colon. Wheatbran is easily available in All-Bran, which can be used as an all-purpose ingredient as well as a breakfast cereal. Here are a few ideas from Kellogg's.

ITALIAN PARMESAN CHICKEN

Serves four

1 cup* Kellogg's All-Bran cereal
1 tbsp plain flour
2 tbsp grated parmesan cheese
2 tsp Italian seasoning
$2\frac{1}{2}$fl.oz (75ml) reduced-calorie
Italian salad dressing

4 boned, skinned chicken breasts
(about 1lb – 500g)
Vegetable oil

In a food processor or with an electric blender process Kellogg's All-Bran cereal, flour, parmesan cheese and Italian seasoning until cereal is in fine crumbs. Place mixture in a shallow dish. Set aside.

Pour salad dressing into a shallow dish. Dip chicken in salad dressing. Coat with cereal mixture. Place in single layer in shallow baking pan coated with oil.

Bake at 350°F/180°C/Gas 4 for about 30 minutes or until tender. Do not cover or turn chicken while baking.

* 1 US cup = 8fl.oz (227 ml)

ORANGE FIG MUFFINS

Makes twelve

1½ cups* plain flour	12 fl.oz (360ml) orange juice
1 tbsp baking powder	1 egg
¼ cup sugar	2 fl.oz (60ml) cup vegetable oil
3 cups Kellogg's Bran Flakes cereal	⅔ cup chopped dried figs
	1 tsp grated orange peel

Stir together flour, baking powder and sugar. Set aside.

Measure Kellogg's Bran Flakes cereal, orange juice, egg, oil, figs, and orange peel into large mixing bowl. Beat well.

Add dry ingredients to cereal mixture, stirring only until combined. Spoon batter evenly into 12 2½ inch (6cm) greased muffin or bun tins.

Bake at 400°F/200°C/Gas 6 for about 25 minutes or until golden brown. Serve warm.

 * 1 US cup = 8fl.oz (227 ml)

JAMBALAYA

Serves eight

½ cup* chopped onions	½ tsp red pepper
¼ cup chopped green pepper	1 bay leaf
16fl.oz (500 ml) reduced-sodium chicken broth	1 cup uncooked long grain rice
14oz (400g) can whole tomatoes	1 cup Kellogg's All-Bran cereal
8 oz (225g) can tomato sauce	½ cup cleaned, whole raw prawns
½ tsp dried basil	2 cups chopped, cooked chicken
½ tsp dried thyme	2 tsp chopped parsley

In a large saucepan combine onions, green pepper, chicken broth, liquid from tomatoes, tomato sauce, herbs and spices. Cook over medium heat, stirring occasionally, until mixture boils.

Chop tomatoes; add to hot mixture along with rice and Kellogg's All-Bran cereal. Cover pan and cook over medium heat until mixture starts to boil. Reduce to simmer and cook 20 minutes longer, stirring occasionally, until rice is tender.

Slice prawns lengthwise into 2 pieces. Add prawns and chicken to rice mixture. Cook 5 minutes longer or until prawns are cooked and chicken is hot. Remove bay leaf and sprinkle with parsley before serving.

* 1 US cup = 8fl.oz (227ml)

HONEY RAISIN BRAN MUFFINS

Makes twelve

1¾ cups* plain flour	10fl.oz (300ml) skimmed milk
1 tbsp baking powder	2½fl.oz (75ml) cup honey
¼ tsp salt (optional)	2 egg whites
2 tbsp sugar	2 fl.oz (60ml) vegetable oil
2½ cups Kellogg's Raisin Bran cereal	

Stir together flour, baking powder, salt and sugar. Set aside.

Measure Kellogg's Raisin Bran cereal, milk and honey into large mixing bowl. Stir to combine. Let stand 3 minutes or until cereal softens.

Add egg whites and oil. Beat well. Add flour mixture, stirring only until combined.

Portion batter evenly into 12 2½ inch (6cm) greased muffin or bun tins.

Bake at 400°F/200°C/Gas 6 for about 20 minutes or until lightly browned. Serve warm.

* 1 US cup = 8fl.oz (227ml)

FIBRE FOR LIFE

The Fibre for Life eating plan recommends that you eat four light meals a day rather than a heavy evening meal that'll be difficult to burn off before you go to bed. Try some of these delicious recipes to get your juices flowing.

MANDARIN AND GRAPE CHEESECAKE

Serves six

Base
2oz (50g) low-fat margarine
2fl.oz (50ml) apple juice
4oz (100g) Kellogg's All-Bran or Bran Buds

Filling
8oz (225g) cottage cheese, seived
5oz (150g) low-fat natural yoghurt
2tbsp lemon juice
1 sachet (11g) gelatine
3fl.oz (75ml) water (hot)
4oz (100g) mandarin oranges
3oz (75g) black grapes

Base

Gently melt the margarine with the apple juice, then stir in the Kellogg's All-Bran or Bran Buds. Press the mixture into the base of a deep 8 inch (20cm) round flan dish.

Topping

Mix the cottage cheese and yoghurt together, and stir in the lemon juice. Set aside.

Dissolve the gelatine in the hot water then quickly stir into the cheese and yoghurt mixture. Mix well together, and place on top of the base.

Allow to set, decorate with the mandarin oranges and the grapes and serve.

CURRANT SWIRL BREAD

Makes one loaf

8oz (225g) bread flour	7fl.oz (200ml) skimmed milk
4oz (100g) wholemeal flour	2oz (50g) low-fat spread
4oz (100g) Kellogg's All-Bran	2 egg whites
1tsp salt	1tsp cinnamon
1 packet dried yeast	2oz (50g) currants
3oz (75g) brown sugar	½oz (15g) granulated sugar

Mix together the different types of flour. Combine ½ of the flour mixture, Kellogg's All-Bran, salt, yeast and 2 tablespoons brown sugar.

In a small saucepan, heat the milk and margarine until warm (120°C–130°C). Gradually add the cereal mixture and mix well together. Add the egg whites and ¼ of the flour mixture and mix well together. Stir in the remaining flour mixture and knead the dough until it is smooth and elastic.

Place the dough in a lightly greased bowl, cover and leave to rise in a warm place until double in volume. Punch down dough and leave to rest for 10 minutes.

Roll dough on lightly floured surface into a $14 \times 8\frac{1}{2}$ inch (35×21cm) rectangle, and wet surface with 1 tablespoon water. Combine the remaining brown sugar and cinnamon. Sprinkle over the wet dough, spread currants evenly over sugar mixture. Starting with shorter side, roll dough lengthwise. Place seam side down in greased 2lb (1kg) loaf tin. Leave to rise until double in size (about 1 hour).

Lightly brush top of bread with 1 tablespoon of milk, sprinkle with granulated sugar. With a sharp knife, make $\frac{1}{8}$ inch (3mm) deep cut lengthwise down centre of loaf.

Bake at 375°F/190°C/Gas 5 for about 30 minutes or until golden brown. Remove from tin and cool on wire.

SWEET & SOUR MEATBALLS

Serves four

4oz (100g) Kellogg's All-Bran	2 egg whites
1½lb (675g) minced beef	10oz (275g) tomato ketchup
2oz (50g) onions, chopped	2tsp Dijon mustard
½tsp salt	1tbsp Worcestershire sauce
¼tsp pepper	10oz (275g) red currant jelly
¼tsp garlic powder	

In a large mixing bowl, stir together the Kellogg's All-Bran, minced beef, onion, salt, pepper, garlic powder and egg whites until thoroughly combined. Shape into 48 1 inch ($2\frac{1}{2}$cm) meatballs, and place in a foil lined shallow baking tray.

Bake at 400°F/200°C/Gas 6 for about 12 minutes or until cooked, drain if necessary.

In a large saucepan, combine remaining ingredients. Bring to the boil, stirring frequently. Place the hot meatballs in the sauce and simmer for 5 minutes. Serve hot.

MIXED FRUIT FLAN

Makes ten portions

8oz (225g) plain flour	1 packet (11g) gelatine
4oz (100g) low-fat spread	12oz (336g) low-fat yoghurt
1oz (25g) brown sugar	4 peaches sliced
4oz (100g) Kellogg's All-Bran, crushed	1 kiwi fruit
4fl.oz (120ml) water	2oz (50g) black cherries
	1 packet red Quick Gel

Put flour into a bowl and rub in the low-fat spread. Stir in the Kellogg's All-Bran, sugar and water and mix into a firm dough.

Roll out and use to line an 8 inch (20cm) round flan dish. Prick base thoroughly with a fork. Bake at 180°C/350°F/Gas 4 for 20 minutes or until cooked, then allow to cool.

Place 3 tablespoons hot water into a pan and sprinkle gelatine on top, stir briskly until thoroughly mixed.

Gradually add the hot gelatine to the yoghurt, stirring constantly. Pour into the cooled crust and refrigerate for about 1 hour or until the yoghurt is set.

Arrange the fruit over the top of the yoghurt. Make up the Quick Gel as instructed on packet, allow to cool slightly, and glaze the tart with the Quick Gel. Allow to set.

ORIENTAL STYLE BEEF AND VEGETABLES

8oz (225g) tin pineapple in natural juice

$\frac{1}{2}$ tsp ginger

1tbsp soy sauce

2 cloves finely chopped garlic

1lb (500g) sirloin steak cut into thin strips

4oz (100g) Kellogg's All-Bran or Bran Buds

1tsp cornflour

1lb (500g) frozen oriental vegetables

2tbsp water

1tbsp vegetable oil

Drain pineapple, reserving juice. Set aside.

In a glass bowl, combine 2 tablespoons pineapple juice, ginger, soy sauce and garlic. Add beef and thoroughly coat with marinade. Cover and refrigerate for 2 hours.

Crush Kellogg's All-Bran or Bran Buds cereal into fine crumbs. Coat beef with cereal. Set aside.

In a small bowl, combine cornflour and remaining pineapple juice, with enough water added to measure 3fl.oz (75ml). Set aside.

In a wok or frying pan, stir-fry vegetables in water for about 3 minutes or until hot and crisp-tender. Remove from wok.

In wok, stir-fry beef in oil until browned. Pour corn-flour mixture over beef and bring to boil, stirring constantly. Add pineapple and vegetables. Return to boil. Serve over hot rice.

APRICOT GLAZED CHICKEN

Serves eight

12oz (336g) jar apricot jam
2tbsp mayonnaise
1tbsp ketchup
1 tsp dry mustard
8 boned skinned chicken breasts
1 tbsp low-fat spread
4oz (100g) finely chopped onions
4oz (100g) finely chopped celery
2oz (50g) mushrooms, sliced

5fl.oz (150ml) chicken stock
5oz (150g) Kellogg's All-Bran or Bran Buds
8oz (225g) chopped water chestnuts
$\frac{1}{2}$ tsp salt
$\frac{1}{4}$ tsp pepper
$\frac{1}{4}$ tsp sage

Combine jam, mayonnaise, ketchup and dry mustard. Set aside for sauce.

Place each chicken breast between waxed paper. Pound to $\frac{1}{8}$ inch (3mm) thickness, being careful not to tear meat. Set aside.

Melt low-fat spread in medium-sized frying pan. Add onions and celery. Stirring frequently, cook over medium heat until crisp-tender. Stir in mushrooms and cook 3–4 minutes longer.

Combine chicken stock and Kellogg's All-Bran or Bran Buds cereal. Let stand for about 1 minute or until cereal absorbs stock. Mix in vegetables, water chestnuts, salt, pepper and sage. Fill each breast with $\frac{1}{4}$ cup filling. Roll, folding ends. Place breasts seam-side down, in a 12×8 inch (30×20cm) shallow baking dish. Cover chicken rolls with reserved sauce.

Bake uncovered at 350°F/180°C/Gas 4, for about 45 minutes or until chicken is tender.

REFERENCES

Eat Better, Live Better, Reader's Digest, 1990

The Food Pharmacy, Jean Carper, Simon and Schuster, 1992

Food Allergy and Intolerance, Brostoff and Gamlin, Bloomsbury, 1990

Mind, Body and Immunity, Rachel Charles, Cedar, 1991

Natures Gift of Food, Jan de Vries, Mainstream, 1992

The Detox Diet, Belinda Grant, Optima, 1991

Fat Chance, Jane Ogden, Routledge, 1992

Irritable Bowel Syndrome, Geoff Watts, Cedar, 1990

The Mediterranean Health Diet, Smith and Goldman, Headline, 1993

REPORTS

'Diets of women with premenstrual syndrome and the effect of changing to a three hourly starch diet', K. Dalton and W.M. Holton, 1992

'Nutrition and the premenstrual syndromes', G.E. Abraham, 1984

'Slimming diets', Bingham, 1987

'The relationship between diet and mental health', Cook and Benton, 1992

'The use of very low calorie diets in obesity', COMA report, 1991

'Dietary fibre and weight loss', C. Bonfield, 1992

'The role of breakfast in diet adequacy of the US population', Morgan et al., 1986

'The relationship between breakfast habits and plasma cholesterol levels in schoolchildren', K. Resnicow, 1991

'The effect of breakfast cereals on short term food intake', Levine et al., 1989

'The role of breakfast cereals in the diets of teenagers aged 16–17 in Britain', H. Crawley, 1993

'Nibbling versus gorging: metabolic advantages of increased meal frequency', D. Jenkins et al., 1989

'An explanation for gallstones in normal weight women: slow intestinal tract', K. Heaton et al., 1993

'Effects of dietary wheatbran fibre on rectal epithelial cell proliferation in patients with resection for colorectal cancer', D.S. Alberts et al., 1990

'Relationship of diet to risk of colorectal adenoma in men', E. Giovannucci et al., 1992

'Dietary fibre and health', Council on Scientific Affairs, 1989

'Dietary fibre and personality factors as determinants of stool output', D. Tucker et al., 1981

'The action of dietary fibre on satiety', V. Burley, 1992

'Dietary reference values for food energy and nutrients for the UK', COMA 1991

'Effect of wheat fibre and vitamins C and E on rectal polyps in patients with familial adenamatous polyposis', J. DeCosse, 1989

'Dietary fibre-mediated mechanisms in carcinogenesis', D. Klurfield, 1991

'Defecation frequency and timing, and stool form in the general population – a prospective study', K. Heaton et al., 1991

'Sources of fibre in the diet of irritable bowel patients prescribed a high-fibre diet', J. Lambert et al., 1992